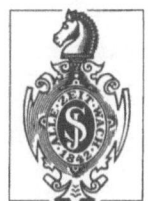

U. Sigwart   G.I. Frank (Eds.)

Coronary Stents

With Contributions by
R.P. Bauman, M. Buchbinder, H. Cabin, B. Cassagneau,
G.D. Chapman, W.D. Edwards, J. Fajadet, D.P. Foley,
G.I. Frank, G.S. Gammon, J. Hirshfeld, D.R. Holmes,
J. Marco, J.G. Murphy, C.A. Pinkerton, G. Robert,
G.S. Roubin, M. Savage, R.A. Schatz, R.S. Schwartz,
P.W. Serruys, U. Sigwart, R.S. Stack, B.H. Strauss,
H.J.C. Swan, P.S. Teirstein, P. Urban, H.M. van Beusekom,
W.J. van der Giessen, M. Vandormael

With 119 Figures and 19 Tables

Springer-Verlag
Berlin Heidelberg New York
London Paris Tokyo
Hong Kong Barcelona
Budapest

ULRICH SIGWART, M.D., FACC, FESC
Royal Brompton National Heart & Lung Hospitals
Sydney Street
London SW3 6NP, UK

GEORGE I. FRANK, M.D.
Cardiovascular Program, Northwest Hospital
1560 North 115th, Suite 206
Seattle, WA 98133, USA

ISBN-13: 978-3-642-76926-9   e-ISBN-13: 978-3-642-76924-5
DOI: 10.1007/978-3-642-76924-5

© Springer-Verlag Berlin Heidelberg 1992
Softcover reprint of the hardcover 1st edition 1992

19/3130 – 5 4 3 2 1 0 – Printed on acid-free paper

Preface

Over the past 15 years, a multitude of new transluminal techniques have been developed, all designed to broaden the range of indications and improve the results of angioplasty. Among these, the implantation of intravascular stents has emerged as the technique with the greatest promise. It has become clear that stenting not only successfully deals with the problem of abrupt closure after angioplasty, but also reduces the incidence of restenosis, the Achilles heel of angioplasty.

The reason why restenosis is reduced may be because the immediate gain of luminal diameter is greater with stenting than with any other technique. Even if the late loss of diameter is similar among most currently used transluminal techniques, the end result will still be better after stenting because of the nearly ideal primary effect.

The aims of this book are twofold: first it presents a state-of-the-art summary of the progress made in stenting so far, and secondly it details some of the prospects for future improvement. The concept of stenting has proved to be a correct one, and therefore all future efforts will be directed towards new, safe, and biologically "friendly" stents.

U. SIGWART
G.I. FRANK

Contents

List of Contributors

R.P. Bauman 155
M. Buchbinder 45
H. Cabin 45
B. Cassagneau 57
G.D. Chapman 155
W.D. Edwards 135
J. Fajadet 57
G.I. Frank 5
D.P. Foley 101
G.S. Gammon 155
J. Hirshfeld 45
D.R. Holmes 135
J. Marco 57
J.G. Murphy 135
C.A. Pinkerton 79

G. Robert 57
G.S. Roubin 79
M. Savage 45
R.A. Schatz 45
R.S. Schwartz 135
P.W. Serruys 101
U. Sigwart 21, 169
R.S. Stack 155
B.H. Strauss 101
H.J.C. Swan 1
P.S. Teirstein 45
P. Urban 21
H.M. van Beusekom 101
W.J. van der Giessen 101
M. Vandormael 57

Coronary Stents – Introduction

H.J.C. SWAN[1]

I admit that I was among the disbelievers when Andrea Grüntzig first demonstrated balloon dilatation for obstructive coronary atherosclerosis. Now, more than a decade later, balloon angioplasty is the most common method for coronary revascularization – at least in the USA. While balloon angioplasty is effective in dilating over 90% of coronary lesions, the overall clinical effectiveness in the long-term management of coronary disease is still unmeasured in comparison with other treatment strategies.

At one end of the spectrum of clinical severity, several randomized trials are underway to compare outcomes in multivessel disease with patients undergoing either PTCA or coronary artery bypass grafting using the internal mammary conduit. At the other end of the spectrum, in patients with mild to moderate symptoms only one small study comparing these two treatment strategies has appeared (Parisi et al., 1992, N. Engl. J. Med. 326:10). The most reasonable interpretation of this study is that adverse "complications" of angioplasty negated the observed increase in exercise treadmill time. The CASS study demonstrated that patients with less severe coronary artery disease may defer revascularization for months, or even years, and then "cross-over" to surgical revascularization. It is logical to assume that for many asymptomatic patients, or those with minimal symptoms, revascularization by coronary angioplasty might also be deferred.

The importance of this consideration relates to the high incidence of delayed restenosis following angioplasty, rather than to primary procedure failure. Between 20% and 40% of patients who undergo coronary angioplasty will experience restenosis – a figure which has not changed in a decade. These figures represent a failure rate which normally would be unacceptable for medical procedures. Lesions at certain locations, including the right coronary osteum, major branch points, and totally occluded vessels, or partially occluded saphenous vein grafts are particularly likely to undergo restenosis. This late "complication" – and it is a major one – raises serious ethical questions for the cardiologist who advised the procedure, or who conducts it. This is particularly important in patients without ischemia and only modest disease angiographically. The early concept of dilatation to

---

[1] 1075 Wallace Ridge, Beverly Hills, CA 90210, USA

Coronary Stents
Edited by U. Sigwart and G.I. Frank
© Springer-Verlag Berlin Heidelberg 1992

"avoid" multivessel disease in later years requires revision in light of our current knowledge of the pathogenesis of atherosclerotic and the resulting clinical syndromes. The claim by many community cardiologists that they "never see important restenosis" and that is "not a problem" has been negated by the leaders in the field. It is to address this currently unanswered dilemma that coronary stents have been introduced, and their development has continued.

The original concept that balloon angioplasty would, in some way, "compress the atherosclerotic lesion in a coronary artery" has proved to be somewhat naive. Clinically important coronary artery disease is usually a longstanding, complex area of vascular disorder. A typical plaque consists of collagen which may be calcified, hypertrophied vascular smooth muscle, thrombus, as well as many lipid elements, each in heterogeneous quantity and distribution. With the exception of cholesterol-rich atherosclerotic plaques, the principle effect of angioplasty is on the more normal and less diseased portion of the target coronary artery with resultant fissuring and splitting of the intima and media. In general, the atherosclerotic portion of the lesion is not greatly changed geometrically, but a form of false aneurysm has been created permitting less obstructed flow.

Many initially questioned the validity of the concept of balloon angioplasty because intravascular ballooning was one of the best ways to produce atherosclerosis in experimental animals. Moreover, damaged or removed vascular endothelium alters the responsiveness of a vessel wall to circulating vasoactive agents causing a degree of vasoconstriction far in excess of what occurs normally, or even under the conditions of vasospasm. Stretching and tearing allows for bleeding within the more normal portions of the vessel wall resulting in both superficial and deep thrombus formation. In this regard balloon angioplasty generally has been ineffective for patients with unstable angina. Primary angioblasty for myocardial infarction has had success but is associated with rethrombosis, particularly following thrombosis. Thus, following balloon angioplasty, a variety of acute changes occur as a consequence of the vascular damage. This may cause acute vasospasm and thrombosis, as well as long-term vascular effects.

At the time of this writing, no treatment form yet employed has substantially affected restenosis. Anticoagulants, antiplatelet agents, thrombolytic agents, beta and calcium channel blocking agents, fish oil, lipid lowering drugs, have all been essentially without effect in reducing the incidence and severity of restenosis. Perhaps a clue comes from the excessive rate of restenosis in patients who have had a suboptimal primary dilatation. This is consistent with the concept that all dilated vessels undergo some degree of "restenosis' as a component of healing which becomes clinically important in a patient with an inadequately dilated vessel. Therefore, the concept of larger balloon diameters, oversizing, and high pressure dilatation maximizes the postdilatation dimension to accommodate any "normal" degree of healing restenosis.

Intravascular stenting – the subject of this text – focuses on the potential role of mechanical devices to provide a practical solution for these continuing problems. Current devices and those which may be developed in the future, have the potential for providing a generous lumen (up to 6 mm) as well as the ability to tack down or resecure an acutely dissected intimal flap. The current metallic devices appear to allow a certain degree of intimal hyperplasia, but usually this does not limit the lumen diameter significantly. However, current devices do exhibit excessive stiffness and limited flexibility. Stent migration, or late perforation of the vessel in which it is inserted, remains a concern. Nonmetallic devices and the incorporation of pharmacologic substances, including growth factor inhibitors, appear to offer significant promise for the future.

Medical device testing is a tedious matter. The problem of restenosis is probably that of overexuberant healing. The application of angioplasty to multivessel coronary disease greatly increases the likelihood of the development of a clinically significant reocclusion in an individual patient. Will stenting become an integral part of the procedure of primary balloon angioplasty, or will it compete for a niche in certain subsets of lesions or patients? In either event, the possible choice of stenting, atherectomy, laser, and ultrasound angioplasty and similar procedures requires a high level of ethical skill and clinical judgement to determine their optimal use in any given clinical situation. This poses a serious practical and ethical dilemma for the community of interventional cardiologists as to who should investigate and ultimately use such devices. Is there any place for the "occasional dilator"? A recent comment on community hospital practice reported "normal coronaries" in 11% of those studied by a cardiology group, but an incidence of 32% by solo practitioners. Such trends underscore the potential for unnecessary intervention. They suggest that appropriate guidelines for angioplasty, and for newer interventions, must be developed as soon as possible and methods for implementation established.

As with any therapy for a complex disorder, an "either/or" approach to the judgement of clinical efficacy is scientifically inappropriate and clinically wrong. In an overall strategy, differing approaches to the multiple subsets – both pathological and temporal – of coronary atherosclerosis properly need to be considered. Balloon angioplasty is being applied to an ever increasing proportion of patients. Superficially, the high primary success and low acute complication rate might suggest that latitude regarding rigorous selection criteria is permissible. I would submit that this is not the case, and attention must be given to the primacy – *do not harm*.

The current text describes the present status of research in intracoronary stenting. The future is speculation. However, in 1980 who could have foreseen the wide (and perhaps at times inappropriate) application of the principal of balloon dilatation over the following decade. In regard to coronary stenting, the carefully collected and honestly documented experience of these dedicated investigators will provide the answers.

Basic Considerations for Coronary Stenting

G.I. Frank[1]

Introduction

Perhaps the most remarkable aspect of coronary angioplasty is not the rate of failure or restenosis, but rather the rate of success. Since the early reports from Grunzig, investigators have consistently achieved long-term patency rates of 70% [1, 2]. The development of new equipment over the years has permitted cardiologists to deal with lesions not possible previously. Better support from guide catheters, more flexible, steerable guide wires, and lower profile balloons have lead to our ability to cross and dilate lesions unapproachable 10 years ago. But the overall success rates at 6 months are largely unchanged. Studies of restenosis continue to report 25%–40% recurrence rates and 3%–5% rates of abrupt closure persist [3, 4].

In the United States today, typically one-half of cases requiring intervention undergo angioplasty, and one-half require bypass surgery. A third of the angioplasty patients return for a repeat procedure within 6 months. Our inability to change these outcomes leads to a huge emotional cost and enormous financial burden for our medical system. Several studies have tried to estimate the relative costs of bypass surgery versus angioplasty as well as the costs of restenosis [5, 6]. Califf et al. made a number of assumptions regarding costs and recurrence rates for angioplasty and bypass surgery [7]. They estimated that $300 million would be saved annually in the USA alone if the restenosis rate could be reduced from 33% to 25%. Additional reductions to 10% or less on a worldwide basis could save billions. Moreover, the human savings would be incalculable. Each physician who has had to explain to a patient that his angioplasty was not successful understands the trauma, anguish, and frustration these words invoke.

This book is devoted to a presentation of a new investigational tool, coronary stents. These devices were developed in response to the problems of abrupt closure and restenosis. In 1986, the first stent was placed by in a human coronary artery [8]. Since then, other stents have been developed

[1] Cardiovascular Program Northwest Hospital, 1560 North 115th, Suite 206, Seattle, WA 98133, USA

Coronary Stents
Edited by U. Sigwart and G.I. Frank
© Springer-Verlag Berlin Heidelberg 1992

and have entered clinical trials. In the subsequent chapters the primary investigators of these stents will present their data and discuss their views for future developments. This chapter will provide background information on the pathophysiology of abrupt closure and restenosis to help explain the relationship of stents to these problems. Some of the clinical factors related to restenosis and other attempts to alter angioplasty results with drug therapy will be discussed.

We hope this book will stimulate clinicians to look forward to the future when a number of these tools will become available for widespread usage. Intracoronary stents and other new interventional tools on the horizon will become part of the armamentarium we all must learn and evaluate for their potential benefits in clinical practice.

Pathophysiology

If cardiologists could visualize microscopically the results of balloon dilatations would they blithely proceed with coronary interventions? When Dotter and Judkins first bougied peripheral vessels with catheters, they believed they were compressing free lipids within an atherosclerotic plaque, forcing the lipid to redistribute within a vessel wall [9]. Animal and human studies, however, have shown that plaques are really composed of non-collapsible fibrocollagenous materials, calcified crystals, and only a small amount of free lipids [10]. It is now clear that balloon dilatations always lead to some disruption of the endothelium and usually cause disruptions, cracks, and tears of the intima and media of the vessel walls (Fig. 1) [11]. The adventitia is almost never affected. Some investigators felt that this trauma would lead to intraluminal and intramedial hemorrhage of the vessel, but this has rarely been observed unless balloon dilatations occur in conjunction with thrombolytic therapy [12]. Animal and human studies suggest that at least 15% of balloon dilatations do not disrupt the media. The normal vessel wall opposite a plaque becomes stretched to provide an enlarged lumen [13]. However, elastic recoil of this normal segment can occur, usually in two to four weeks, and lead to a recurrent ischemic lesion. These observations possibly explain clinical reports that small dissections induced at the time of angioplasty are harbingers for lower rates of restenosis [14].

Abrupt vessel closures probably are caused by large flaps of the intima that fold over to compromise the vessel lumen. In many cases thrombus forms due to the decreased flow. There may be a component of coronary spasm, possibly initiated by the damaged vessel wall itself [15, 16].

Unfortunately, we don't have mechanisms which allow us to see directly the results of balloon dilatations at the level of the vessel wall. If we had this capability, we might be able to choose a therapy or further intervention based upon these findings. Angioscopy has been available as a research tool

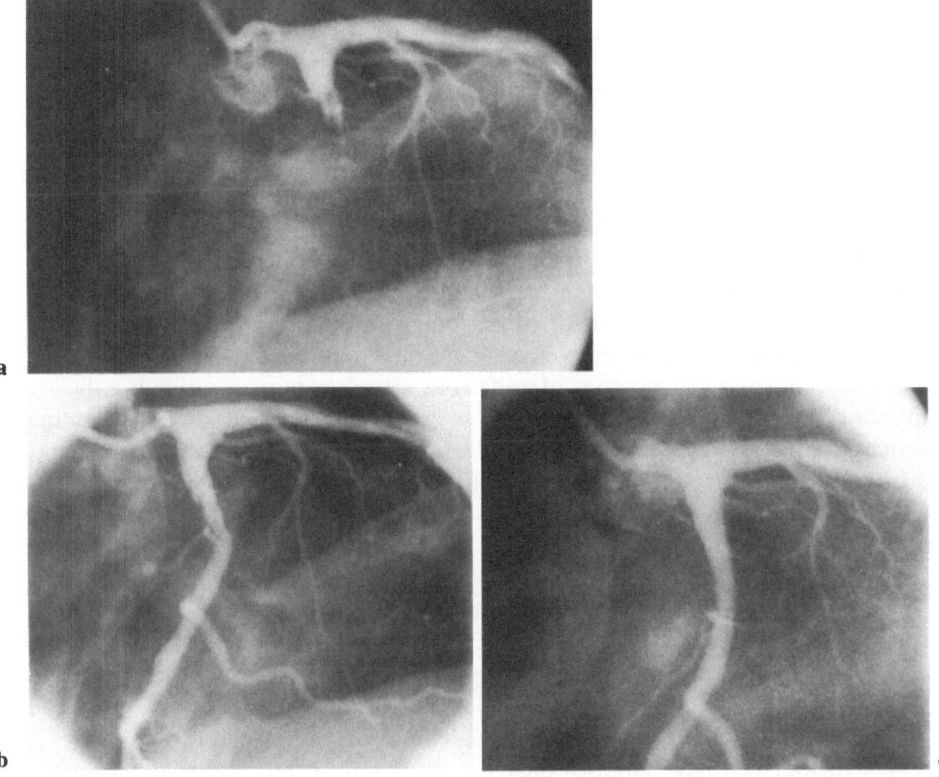

Fig. 1. a Patient with unstable angina and severe lesion involving the circumflex artery.
b Appearance after unsuccessful angioplasty, including prolonged, low pressure inflations.
c After placing a Medinvent self-expanding stent

over the past several years. Initially only large proximal lesions could be seen. New equipment now permits visualization of smaller, distal vessels, including those around bends [17]. New optics have also been developed which should permit better discrimination of the appearance of thrombus from intimal flaps and other abnormalities [18]. This tool is likely to remain an investigative device, however, until its clinical usefulness is clearly established.

Recently, Waller presented his findings which correlated the angiographic appearance of lesions after balloon angioplasty with the microscopic appearance seen at autopsies [19]. He analyzed 76 angioplasty sites from 66 patients. Ten sites (14%) were described at the time of the procedure as "smooth appearing." Microscopic examination showed that 8 of these sites had eccentric plaques without any evidence of intimal-medial injury, and two sites had shallow, minimal intimal disruptions. Intraluminal haziness was seen at 29 locations (38%) which correlated with the presence of intimal injuries in 9 locations and intimal-medial tears in 19 locations. One site had a tear involving the intima and media with the presence of thrombus layering along the wall. Intimal flaps were noted by the angiographers at 33 sites (43%). Twenty-nine of these areas demonstrated deep intimal disruptions, and 4 sites had deep intimal disruptions extending into the media. In the procedure where the cardiologists saw a large dissection, a deep intimal-medial tear was seen extending longitudinally through the media at autopsy. Waller's report suggests that we may be able to derive significant information regarding changes in the vessel wall from angiography alone. This knowledge could allow a future cardiologist to make decisions regarding the need for other interventions, and the choice of such an intervention, based on the vessel wall abnormality.

The physiological process of repairing intracoronary injuries involves a number of steps, of which only some are well understood. The healing process appears to be initiated by the presence of platelets which are recruited to the injured area by different factors. Platelet membrane receptors interact with adhesive glycoproteins, subendothelial microfibrils, collagen, and other proteins [20]. The platelets deposit along the subendothelial surface releasing other agonists that stimulate further platelet aggregation. These agonists include ADP, serotonin, thromboxane A_2, and PDGF (platelet derived growth factor). PDGF is thought to be the prime factor which recruits smooth muscle cells from the intima and media and leads to their hyperplastic response [21]. Blood-borne monocytes are also recruited at an injury site and release MDGF (IL-1, monoctye derived growth factor), which further activates smooth muscle cell proliferation. Deep injury to the vessel wall can activate the coagulation system via both the intrinsic and the extrinsic pathways generating thrombin, which in turn catalyzes the conversion of fibrinogen to fibrin [22].

This healing process stops 70% of the time, leaving a smooth vessel wall with good flow and no significant luminal narrowing. In 30% of angioplasties the process continues unchecked, eventually leading to fibrocellular hyperplasia with the smooth muscle cell as the primary cell type [23]. The control mechanisms for this response are still unclear and are an area of very active research. Investigators have examined the possibility that drugs might limit the fibrocellular hyperplasia. The approach has involved anticoagulant drugs, anti-inflammatory drugs, and antimitotic agents. Calcium blocking drugs have also been studied in the hopes that at least part of the mechanism of restenosis involves coronary spasm [24]. In the next section we'll review the results of the more important drug studies.

Pharmacological Therapy for Abrupt Closure and Restenosis

One of the earliest drugs studied for its effect on abrupt closure and restenosis was aspirin. Aspirin blocks platelet production of thromboxane A_2

in low doses that are clinically well tolerated [25]. Studies have shown definite reductions in the incidence of acute myocardial infarction post angioplasty with various doses of aspirin [26]. Ticlopidine, another agent which alters platelet function, has also been effective in reducing the incidence of myocardial infarction associated with angioplasty [27]. The use of dipyridamole in conjunction with aspirin has not shown any additional benefit [28]. No study has been able to demonstrate that any of these antiplatelet regimens effect restenosis [29]. This group of antiplatelet drugs do not slow platelet deposition on the subendothelial surface and they do not alter the release of PDGF. These factors may explain their lack of effect on restenosis.

Heparin has been shown in experimental studies to be an important adjunct to the angioplasty procedure. In patients with unstable angina and those patients who have received thrombolytic therapy for acute myocardial infarction, heparin therapy for 1–8 days prior to angioplasty decreases the incidence of acute occlusion [30, 31]. Heparin also decreases the smooth muscle cell response to vessel wall injury in animal models [32]. This finding stimulated studies to determine if heparin could lower the rates of restenosis. In two studies heparin was administered for 18–24 h post angioplasty [33] or for 36 h post angioplasty and did not lower the rate of restenosis (Dr. Budge Smith, personal communication).

Other anticoagulants will be studied in the future for their effects on acute closure and possibly restenosis. Hirudin, which was initially found in the salivary glands of medical leeches and can now be made by recombinant DNA techniques, holds considerable promise. It not only effects platelet function, but also appears to prevent platelet deposition along an injured vessel wall. Investigators are presently examining the potential benefits of monoclonal antibodies against platelet membrane receptors. In animal models these agents are more effective than aspirin. They alter platelet function and limit platelet deposition along the subendothelial surface of injured vasculature [34].

The ability of anti-inflammatory drugs to limit the smooth muscle cell response to injury also has been evaluated in two separate studies [35, 36]. Corticosteroids in high doses showed no definite effect on restenosis rates. Further investigations will likely pursue the potential benefits of anti-inflammatory agents as well as antimitotic drugs. Until more specific knowledge of the control mechanisms of smooth muscle cell hyperplasia are known, these classes of agents seem very appealing teleologically.

Several studies have evaluated the effects of calcium blocking agents on the incidence of restenosis [37, 38]. There have been no clear-cut benefits demonstrated either acutely or long-term. Despite these findings, it's common practice to prescribe these agents after angioplasty, which only adds to the cost of the procedure.

Omega-3 fatty acids caught the public eye after reports that populations who consumed large amounts had a substantially lower incidence of atherosclerosis. This substance also has effects on the clotting mechanism and possibly has additional properties which are not well understood [39]. Five different studies have been published which examined the effects of omega-3 fatty acids on restenosis. Three studies have shown benefits of varying degrees [40–42], and two studies have demonstrated no significant change [43, 44]. Further evaluation of this food supplement is necessary before we can make any definite statements regarding its possible benefit.

Thus far, no single agent, or combination of agents, has shown any definite effect on restenosis. Combinations of anti-inflammatory and anti-mitotic drugs in significant doses which might have effects on smooth muscle cell hyperplasia are contraindicated due to their systemic toxicity. Newer delivery methods which can instill drugs directly at the vessel wall will be studied in the future for their potential benefit and decreased toxicity. The possibility of injecting an agent directly into a vessel wall, at an area of exuberant smooth muscle cell proliferation, may be part of our approach to this disease in the future. It's quite likely that one agent, or combination of agents, will be given with mechanical interventions to decrease restenosis successfully. Coronary stents hold considerable promise in this regard. They are an indwelling device which could be used to deliver a drug directly at the site of intimal proliferation, either acutely or over an extended period of time.

Coronary Stents

Preliminary data suggests that the initial success of balloon dilatations may be related to limiting vessel wall damage and maintaining good flow. Some investigators working with animal models have shown that small amounts of endothelial damage do not lead to smooth muscle cell hyperplasia [45]. Other animal research has demonstrated that maintenance of normal flow also appears to restrict the smooth muscle cell response [46]. If we could replace the diseased vessel segment with new material that was smooth and nonthrombogenic and maintained normal flow, the problems of restenosis might be solved. Coronary stents provide a partial solution. They are a support structure, "tacking up" damaged intima, and maintaining normal flow through a diseased vascular segment which may prove to be the most important aspect in the control mechanisms of intimal hyperplasia. The process of endothelialization covers the stent so that it is not a continuous nidus for clot formation.

The Histology of Coronary Stents

Dotter demonstrated in his initial report that implanted stents which re-mained free of thrombus also remained patent [47]. When the animals were

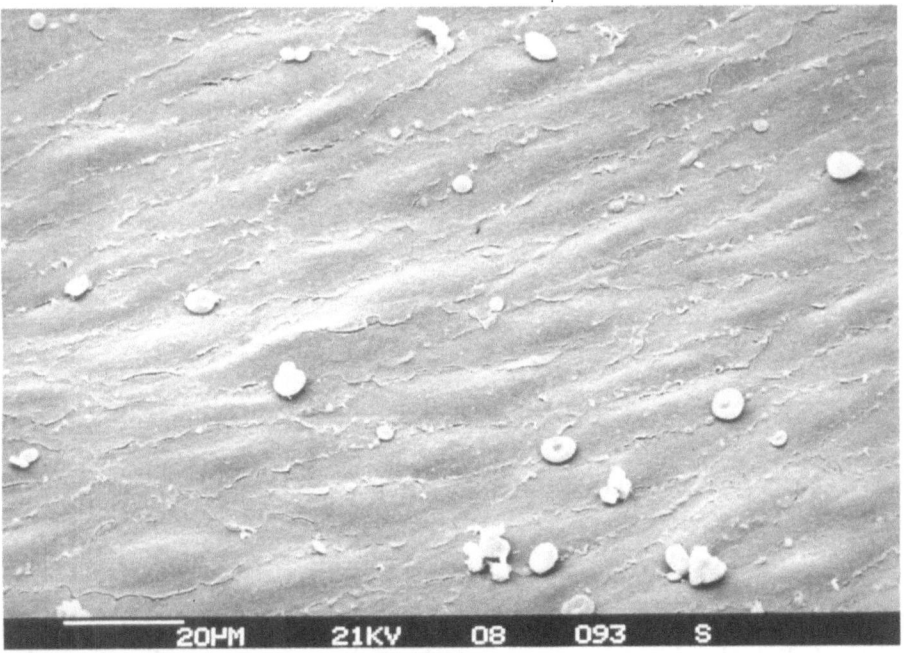

Fig. 2. Electron microscopy of neoendothelium covering a stent 9 months after coroanry implantation in a dog

sacrificed, these devices were firmly embedded into the vessel wall and were covered by normal-appearing endothelium. Since these early observations by Dotter, a number of different studies have reported the pathological response to different materials and stent designs in various animal models. Regardless of the animal model, the initial tissue response observed was the deposition of a fine layer of platelets and fibrin along the stent surface [48, 49]. In time, neointima formed, and the foreign body became fully covered with a layer of new endothelium (Fig. 2). The time for complete endothelialization varied between 2 weeks in rabbits and 3 months in guinea pigs [50]. In these studies, all side branches covered by the stents remained patent (Fig. 3).

The process of endothelialization is affected by a number of different factors. If a metal strut is too thick, it can slow and sometimes stop endothelialization completely. Small stents are much more likely to become involved with thrombus and occlude prematurely. The size of the pores of a stent are significant [51]. The process of endothelialization occurs not only from both ends of the device, but also through the pores themselves. The type of material used to form the stent plays a significant role [52]. Many investigators have felt that negatively charged materials would be superior because blood-borne elements are negatively charged and might be less

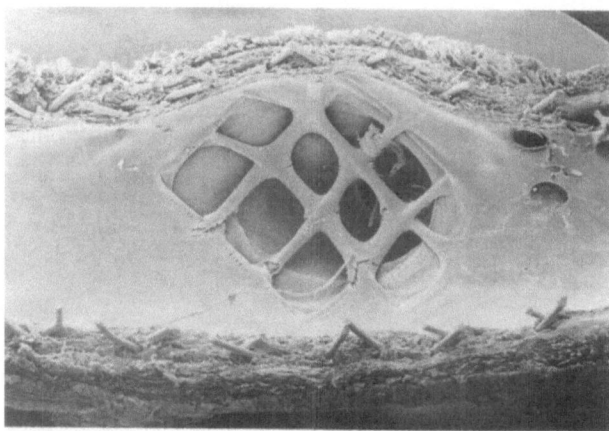

Fig. 3. Scanning electron micrograph of self-expanding stent in a dog's femoral artery. Side branch orifice covered by the stent is patent. (Reprinted with permission)

likely to deposit on a similarly charged surface. Most metals are negatively charged, but also highly corrosive, making them unsuitable for these devices. Up until now, the most widely used material for stents has been highly polished stainless steel. However, polymers, some of which are biodegradable, are now being studied in animal models and may well represent the primary material for future research efforts. Two chapters of this book are devoted to these new materials.

The History of Stents

Dotter's initial experiments in the 1960's with stents involved the use of both plastic tubing and stainless steel coilspring prostheses which he implanted into the peripheral vessels of dogs [45]. The impervious plastic tube grafts all clotted within 24 h and were not studied further. The stainless steel coilspring design did not clot when heparin was administered during the first 4 days after placement, and it became the standard for subsequent design efforts.

Several investigators examined variations of the metal coil design made from stainless steel or from nitinol [53, 54]. Nitinol is a temperature-dependent, memory-shaped, nickel and titanium alloy. Nitinol stents are appealing since they allow "automatic" expansion once they are positioned in the vessel and assume body temperature. However, they require refrigeration before deployment and therefore are quite cumbersome. These studies demonstrated that more closely woven stent designs tended to have greater thrombogenicity, probably because more metal was involved for a

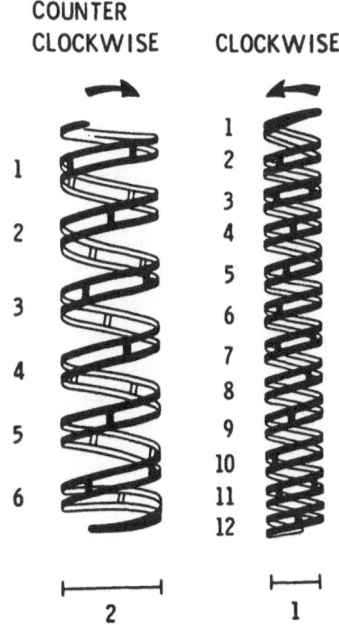

Fig. 4. Double helix stent described by Maass et al. in 1983 [55]. (Reprinted with permission)

given length of stented vessel. Moreover, small diameter stents were more likely to clot than larger devices.

In 1983 Maass et al. described the experimental use of several different self-expanding stents that could be stretched onto an introducing device and released into the vascular lumen where they expanded due to their elastic properties [55]. Some of these stents had problems with both migration and thrombosis. The "double helix" stent configuration (Fig. 4) proved more stable [56]. The investigators did not observe migration or occlusive thrombus formation with this design. At the time of autopsy there was no evidence of pressure necrosis and endothelialization was completed within 6 weeks of implantation. However, the stent required a bulky introducing system which made it unsuitable for small arteries. All these stents were made from surgical stainless steel and were configured as either wire of 0.3–0.5 mm diameter, or metal bands of 0.08–0.30 mm thick and 1.5 mm wide.

Several of the initial problems of self-expanding stents were solved when the coil model was replaced with a mesh configuration composed of interwoven strands of 0.06 or 0.08 mm surgical stainless steel (Fig. 5). The design was suggested by Dr. Sigwart and developed by the Medinvent Company of Switzerland. This device was the first used in human trials and has been studied extensively over the past 4 years [8]. These results will be discussed in detail in the next chapter.

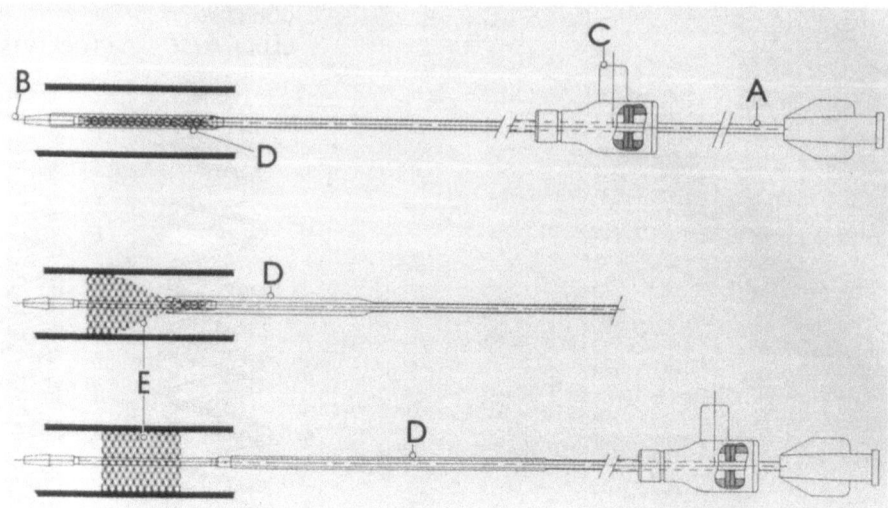

Fig. 5. Schematic representation of self-expanding stent and introducing system. *A*, Central shaft; *B*, guide wire; *C*, inflation port; *D*, constraining membrane; *E*, stent

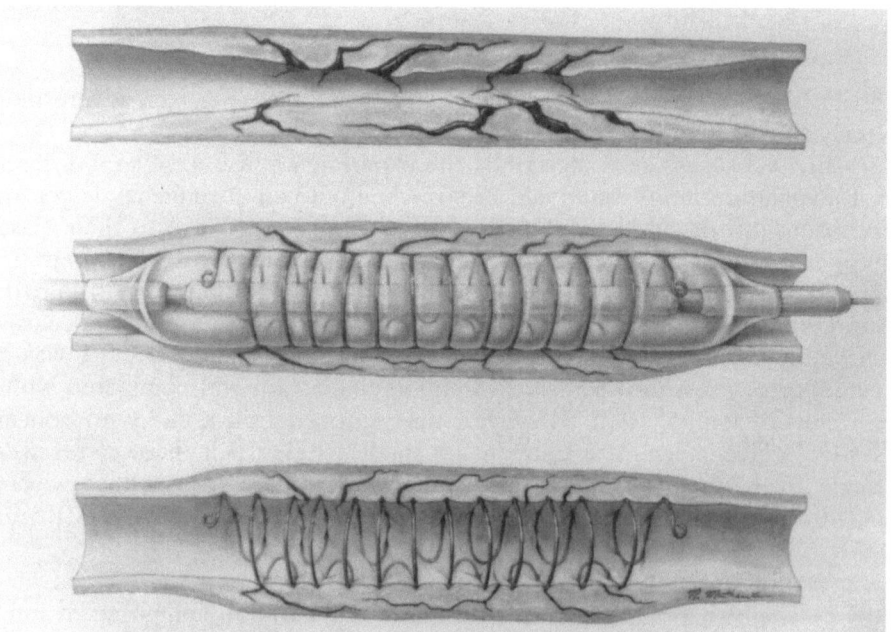

Fig. 6. Diagrammatic representation of the Gianturco-Roubin balloon-expandable stent (reprinted with permission)

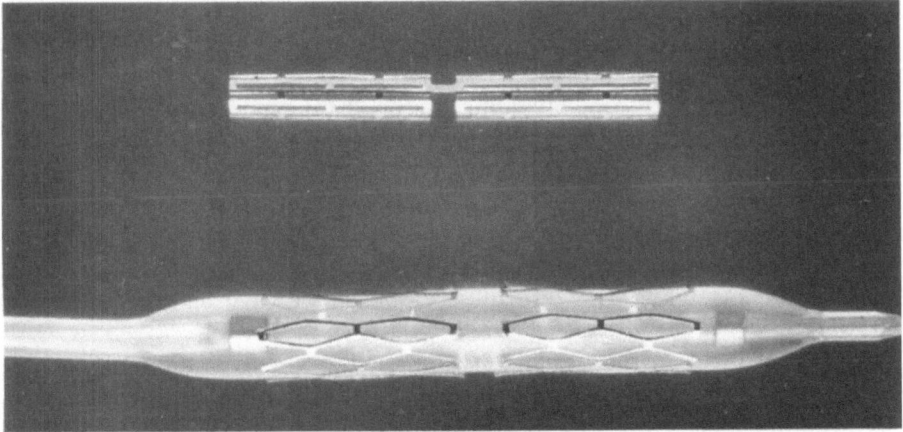

Fig. 7. Palmaz–Schatz balloon-expandable stent (reprinted with permission)

Several other variations from the early stent designs have been used in clinical trials. The group at Emory has studied the Gianturco-Roubin stent in situations of abrupt closure and are now investigating its role as a permanent implantable device (Fig. 6) [57]. This device represents a variation of Dotter's original coiled spring design. The stent is made from a monofilament of 150 mm stainless steel and is compressed onto an angioplasty balloon. The maximum diameter of the stent is determined by the balloon size at maximum inflation. A chapter in the book is devoted to this "balloon expandable" appliance. The other design which has undergone significant clinical investigation is the Palmaz–Schatz stent (Fig. 7) [58]. This device is also balloon-expandable. In its resting state, the stent appears to be rectangular stainless steel boxes which are interconnected by a stainless steel rod. The rod, which represents a modification by Schatz of the original Palmaz design, provides some flexibility for the device [59]. When expanded, the rectangles assume a diamond shaped configuration which provides structural strength to help avoid vessel wall recoil. Two chapters in the book are devoted to discussing this stent's role in abrupt closure and prevention of restenosis.

Conclusion

As you read the chapters in this book and evaluate the results of these early studies on coronary stents, keep in mind that these devices represent an initial design to overcome the major complications of balloon dilatation procedures. The data represents the results from the first iteration of these devices which usually were inserted under difficult circumstances where angioplasty failure, or restenosis, had already occurred. Despite this set of adverse circumstances, the data shows that stents are very effective in situations of abrupt closure, avoiding the need for emergency surgery [55]. Studies also demonstrate that stents can reduce the rate of restenosis [8]. All of these devices were extensively studied in lab animals before clinical trials. However, the reaction of an animal's iliac artery is certainly not the same as a human coronary diseased with atherosclerosis. Unexpected complications occurred once clinical trials were initiated. Early occlusion from thrombosis, embolization of stents, and difficulty in placement have all been reported [60, 61].

Major changes in the designs of stents will occur over the next several years. The newer devices should prove easier to deploy, radiopaque, and nonthrombogenic. They will be flexible enough to go around curves into small distal beds, but stiff enough to prevent elastic recoil of the vessel wall. The stent probably will serve as a means for delivering drugs directly to the vessel wall. Hopefully, the success of intracoronary stents and other new devices under investigation will extend the indications for angioplasty, decrease the rates for emergency surgery, and insure much better long-term patency rates.

Acknowledgements. My wife, Joan, was invaluable as a critic and editor of this manuscript. Dr. Ulrich Sigwart gave me his time and ideas regarding intracoronary stents which was an enormous help. This work was supported by grants from Northwest Hospital Foundation and Advanced Cardiovascular Systems.

References

1. Holmes DR Jr, Vliestra RE, Smith HC et al. (1984) Restenosis after percutaneious transluminal coronary angioplasty (PTCA): a report from the PTCA Registry of the National Heart, Lung, and Blood Institue. Am J Cardiol 53 [Suppl]:77c–81c
2. Nobuyoshi M, Kimura T, Nosaka H, Mioka S, Ueno K, Yokoi H, Hamasaki N, Horiuchi H, Ohishi H (1988) Restenosis after successful percutaneous transluminal coronary angioplasty: serial angiographic follow-up of 229 patients. J Am Coll Cardiol 12:616–623
3. Ellis SG, Roubin GS, King SB, Douglas JS, Weintraub WS, Thomas RG, Cox WR (1988) Angiographic and clinical predictors of acute closure after native vessel coronary angioplasty. Circulation 77:372–379
4. Detre K, Holubkov PH, Kelsey S, Cowley M, Kent K, Williams D et al. (1988) Percutaneous transluminal coronary angioplasty in 1985–1986 and 1977–1981. N Engl J Med 318:265–270
5. Reeder GS, Krishan I, Nobrega FT, Naessus J, Christianson JB et al. (1984) Is percutaneous transluminal angioplasty less espensive than bypass surgeryr? N Engl J Med 311:1157–1162
6. Black AJR, Roubin GS, Sutor C, Moe N, Jarboe JM, Douglas JS, King SB III (1988) Comparative costs of percutaneous transluminal angioiplasty and coronary bypass grafting in multivessel coronary artery disease. Am J Cardiol 62:809–811

7. Califf RM et al. (1990) Restenosis: The clinical issues. In: Topol EJ (ed) Textbook of interventional cardiology. Saunders, Philadelphia, p 372
8. Sigwart U, Puel J, Mirkovitch V, Joffre F, Kappenberger L (1987) Intravascular stents to prevent occlusion and restenosis after transluminal angiopolasty. N Engl J Med 316:701–706
9. Dotter CT, Judkins MP (1964) Transluminal treatment of atherosclerotic obstruction: description of a new technique and preliminary report of its application. Circulation 30:654–660
10. Sanborn TA, Faxon DP, Waugh MD, Small DM, Haudenschild CC, Gottsman SB, Ryan TJ (1982) Transluminal angiioplasty in experimental atherosclerosis. Circulation 66:917–922
11. Waller BF, Gorfinkel HJ, Rogers FJ, Kent KM, Roberts WC (1984) Early and late morphological changes in major epicardial coronary arteries after percutaneous transluminal angioplasty. Am J Cardiol 53:42c–47c
12. Waller BF, Rothbaum DA, Pinkerton CA, Cowley MJ, Linnemeier TJ, Orr C, IRons M, Helmuth RA, Willis ER, Aust C (1987) Status of the myocardium and infarct-related coronary artery in 19 necropsy patients with acute recanalization using pharmacologic, mechanical or combined types of reperfusion therapy. J Am Coll Cardiol 9:785–801
13. Waller BF (1985) Coronary luminal shape and the arc of desease free wall: morphologic observations and clinical relevance. J Am Coll Cardiol 6:1100–1101
14. Matthews BJ, Ewels CJ, Kent KM (1988) Coronary dissection: a predictor of restenosis? Am Heart J 115:547–554
15. Sinclair IN, McCabe CH, Sipperly ME, Baim DS (1988) Predictors, therapeutic options and long-term outcome of abrupt reclosure. Am J Cardiol 61:615–665
16. Baim DS, Ignatius EJ (1988) Use of percutaneous transluminal coronary agioplasty: results of a current survey. Am J Cardiol 61:3G–8G
17. Smith P, Prevosti L, Underhill D, Leon M (1989) Basic principles of operation and performance cahracteristics. In: White GH, White RA (eds) Angioscopy: vascular and coronary applications. Year Book Medical Publishers, Chicago, pp 6–19
18. Johnson C, Hansen DD, Vracko R, Ritchie J (1989) Angioscopy – more sensitive than for identifying thrombus, distal emboli and sunbintimal dissection. J Am Coll Cardiol 13:146A
19. Waller BF (1988) Morphologic correlates of coronary angiographic patterns at the site of percutaneous transluminal coronary angioplasty. Clin Cardiol 11:817–823
20. Hawiger J (1987) Formation and regulation of platelet and fibrin hemostatic plug. Hum Pathol 18:111–122
21. Ross R (1986) The pathogenesis of atherosclerosis – an update. N Engl J Med 314:488–500
22. Fuster V, Badimon L, Cohoen M et al. (1988) Insights into the pathogenesis of acute ischemic syndromes. Circulation 77:1213–1220
23. Liu MW, Roubin GS, King SB (1989) Restenosis after coronary angioplasty. Potential biologic determinants and role of intimal hyperplasia. Circulation 79:1374–1387
24. Hollman J, Austin GE, Gruentzig AR (1983) Coronary artery spasm at the site of angioplasty in the first two months after successful PTCA. J Am Coll Cardiol 2:1039–1045
25. Oates JA, Fitzgerald GA, Branch RA, Jackson EK, Knapp HR, Roberts LJ (1988) Clinical implications of prostaglandin and thromboxane A_2 formation (first of two parts). N Engl J Med 319:691–698
26. Barnatham ES, Schwartz JS, Taylor L et al. (1987) Aspirin and dipyridamole in the prevention of acute coronary thrombosis complicating coronary angioplasty. Circulation 76:125–134
27. White CW, Chaitman B, Lassar TA et al. (1987) Antiplatelet agents are effective in reducing the immediate complications of PTCA: results from the ticlopidine multicenter trial (abstract). Circulation 76 [Suppl IV]:1–400

28. Barnatham ES, Schwartz JS, Taylor L et al. (1987) Aspirin and dipyridamole in the prevention of acute coronary thrombosis complicating coronary angioplasty. Circulation 76:125–134
29. Schwartz L, Bourassa MG, Lesperance J et al. (1988) Aspirin and dirpyridamole in the prevention of restenosis after percutaneous transluminal coronary angiopalsty. N Engl J Med 318:1714–1719
30. Lukas MA, Deutsch E, Laskey WK (1988) Beneficial effects of heparin therapy on PTCA outcome in unstabel angina (abstr). J Am Coll Cardiol II [Suppl]:132A
31. Pow TK, Varrichione TR, Jacobs AK et al. (1988) Does pretreatment with heparin prevent abrupt closure following PTCA? (Abstract). J Am Coll Cardiol II [Suppl]:238A
32. Clowes AW, Karnowsky MJ (1987) Suppression by heparin of smooth muscle cell proliferation in injured arteries. Nature 265:625–626
33. Ellis SG, Roubin GS, Wilentz J et al. (1989) Effect of 18–24 hour heparin administration for prevention of restenosis after uncomplicated coronary angioplasty. Am Heart J 117:777–782
34. Badimon L, Badimon JJ, Chesebro JH et al. (1988) Inhibition of thrombus formation: blockage of adhesive glycoprotein mechanisms versus blockage of the cyclooxygenase pathway (abstract). J Am Coll Cardiol II [Suppl A]:30A
35. Hartzler GO, Rutherford BD, McConahay DR, Johnson WI, Calkins MM (1987) High-dose steroids for prevention of recurrent restenosis in post-PTCA: a randomized trial (abstract). J Am Coll Cardiol 9:185A
36. Pepine CJ, Hirshfield JW, MacDonald RG et al. (1988) A controlled trial of corticosteroids to prevent restenosis following coronary angioplasty (abstract). Circulation 78:II–291
37. Corcos T, David PR, Val PG, Renkin J et al. (1985) Failure of deltiazem to prevent restenosis after percutaneous transluminal coronary angioplasty. Am Heart J 109:926–931
38. Whitworth HB, Roubin GS, Hollman J et al. (1986) effect of nifedipine recurrent stenosis after percutaneous transluminal coronary angioplasty. J Am Coll Cardiol 8:1271–1276
39. Leaf A, Weber PC (1988) Cardioivascular effects of n-3 fatty acids. N Engl J Med 318:549–557
40. Milner MR, Gallino RA, Leffingwell A et al. (1988) High dose Omega-3 fatty acid supplementation reduces clinical restenosis after coronary angioplasty (abstract). Circulation 78:II–634
41. Dehmer GJ, Popma JJ, van den Berg EK et al. (1988) Reduction in the rate of early restenosis after coronary angiioplasty by a diet supplemented with n-3 fatty acids. N Engl J Med 319:733–740
42. Slack OD, Van Tassel J, Orr CM et al. (1987) Can oral fish oil supplement minimize restenosis after percutaneous coronary angioplasty (abstract)? J Am Coll Cardiol 9:64A
43. Grigg LE, Kay TWH, Valentine PA et al. (1989) Determinants of restenosis and lack of effect of dietary supplementation with eicosapentaenoic acid on the incidence of coronary artery restenosis after angioplasty. J Am coll Cardiol 13:665–672
44. Reis GS, Sipperly ME, Boucher TM et al. (1988) Results of a randomized, double-blind placebo – controlled trial of fish oil for prevention of restenosis after PTCA (abstract). Circulation 78:II–291
45. Tada T, Reidy MA (1985) Endothelial regeneration, IX. Arterial injury followed by rapid endothelial repair induces smooth muscle cell proliferation but not intimal thickening. Am J Pathol 118:173–177
46. Haudenschild C, Studer A (1971) Early interactions between blood cells and severely damaged rabbit aorta. Eur J Clin Invest 2:1–7
47. Dotter CT (1969) Transluminally-placed coilspring endarterial tube grafts. Invest Radiol 4:329–332

48. Roubin GS, Robinson KA, King SB et al. (1987) Early and late results of intracoronary arterial stenting after coronary angioplasty in dogs. Circulation 76:891–897
49. Palmaz JC, Windeler SA, Garcia F et al. Atherosclerotic rabit aortal: expandable intraluminal grafting. Radiology 160:723–726
50. Steele PM, Chesebro JH, Stanson A et al. (1985) Balloon angioplasty: natural history of the pathophysiological response to injury in a pig model. Circ Res 57:105–112
51. Wright KC, Wallace S, Charnsangavej C et al. (1985) Percutaneous endovascular stents: an experimental evaluation. Radiology 156:69–72
52. Baier RE, Dutton RC (1969) Initial events in interaction of blood with a foreign surface. J Biomed Mater Res Symp 3:191–193
53. Dotter CT, Buschmann RW, McKinney MK, Roesch J (1983) Transluminal expandable nitinol stent grafting: preliminary report. Radiology 147:259–260
54. Cragg A, Lund G, Rysavy J et al. (1983) Nonsurgical placement of arterial endoprostheses: a new technique using nitinol wire. Radiology 147:261–263
55. Maass D, Demierre D, Deaton D et al. (1983) Transluminal implantation of self-adjusting expandable prosthesis: principals, techniques and results. Prod Artif Org 27:979–987
56. Maass D, Zollokofer CL, Lorgioder F, Senning A (1984) Radiological follow-up of transluminally inserted vascular endoprothesis: an experimental study using expanding spiral prosthesis. Radiology 150:659–663
57. Roubin GS, Douglas JS, Lembo NJ et al. (1988) Intracoronary stenting for acute closure following percutaneous transluminal coronary angioplasty (abstract). Circulation 78 [Suppl]:II–407
58. Palmaz JC (1988) Balloon – expandable intravascular stents. Am J Radiol 150:1263–1269
59. Schatz RA (1988) A view of vascular stents. Circulation 79:445–457
60. Schatz RA, Leon MB, Baim DS et al. (1989) Balloon – expandable intracoronary stents: initial results of a multicenter study (abstract). Circulation 80:II–174
61. Serruys PW, Beatt KJ, van der Giessen WJ (1989) Stenting of coronary arteries. Are we the sorcere's apprentice? Eur Heart J 10:774–782

The Self-Expanding Mesh Stent

P. Urban[1] and U. Sigwart[2]

Mechanisms of Action and Limitations of Angioplasty

Percutaneous transluminal coronary angioplasty has developed at a rapid pace over the 13 years since its introduction. As experience has grown, the indications for its use have greatly expanded [1–5]. Today, PTCA compares favorably with coronary artery bypass surgery in terms of symptom relief, patient discomfort [6], cost [7], and rates for returning to work [8]. The procedure has reached such a level of success that randomized studies comparing angioplasty to either bypass surgery or medical treatment are now, appropriately, underway [9].

Despite improvements in technical equipment and the growing experience of operators, the two major limitations of balloon angioplasty persist unchanged. Abrupt postangioplasty closure complicates 5% of procedures [10], and restenosis occurs in 30%–40% of patients [11–14]. One mechanical device, the coronary stent, shows promise for modifying the rates of both acute occlusion and restenosis. Stents provide a "scaffolding" to support the vessel wall, tack down intimal flaps, smooth the luminal surface improving blood flow, and prevent vessel wall recoil. In 1986, the self-expanding mesh stent was the first of these devices deployed in a coronary vessel [15]. Over the past 4 years, we have examined the role of the self-expanding mesh stent (Fig. 1) under circumstances of abrupt closure [16], restenosis of native coronary vessels [17], and restenosis of bypass graft vessels [18]. The self-expanding mesh stent has also been studied by others around the world. This chapter will describe the results of these investigations.

Histology

Experimental evidence from several different animal studies shows that a thin fibrin and platelet layer is deposited on a stent within minutes following

[1] Cardiology Center, University Hospital, 1211 Geneva 4, Switzerland
[2] Royal Brompton National Heart and Lung Hospital, Sydney Street, London SW3 6NP, Great Britain

Coronary Stents
Edited by U. Sigwart and G.I. Frank
© Springer-Verlag Berlin Heidelberg 1992

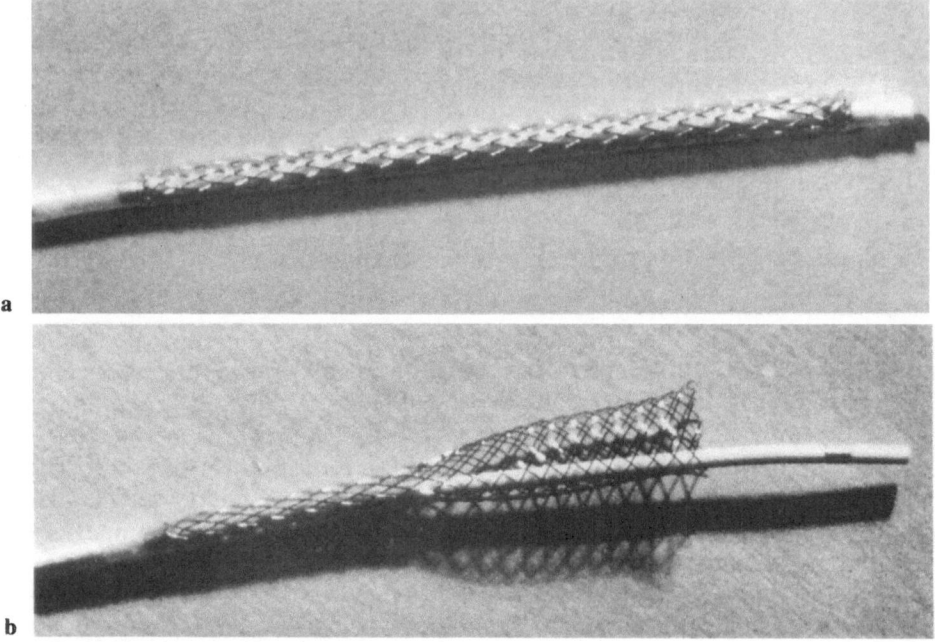

Fig. 1a,b. Self-expanding stent (**a**) constrained on balloon and (**b**) partially deployed as constraining membrane is slowly removed

implantation [19–22]. The stent slowly becomes embedded in thickened intima and the endoluminal surface is eventually covered by neoendothelium. The neoendothelial covering is completed within 1–8 weeks, depending on the type of stent and the animal model studied. Using a balloon-expandable stent in the rabbit model, Palmaz et al. [23] observed an immature endothelial cover with a "crazy-paving" appearance after 1 week, and normal-appearing endothelium with flat, elongated cells at 8 weeks (Fig. 2). Using the same stent deployed in a dog's peripheral artery, these investigators observed that the development of neoendothelium took 3 weeks [24].

Rousseau and others have made similar observations with the self-expanding stent [15, 19]. They inserted 47 stents in dogs and sheep and noted a thin fibrin and platelet layer over the stent within the first few hours of deployment. Complete endothelial covering was observed at 3 weeks. The rapidity of the endothelial coating was probably due to the mesh design which allowed islands of endothelium to grow between the stainless steel strands and eventually coalesce. The thickness of the neointima varied between 50 and 500 μm. Pressure necrosis was not seen, but thinning and slight fibrosis of the underlying media was observed with all stent devices [20, 23]. All side-branches covered by stents remained patent (Fig. 3).

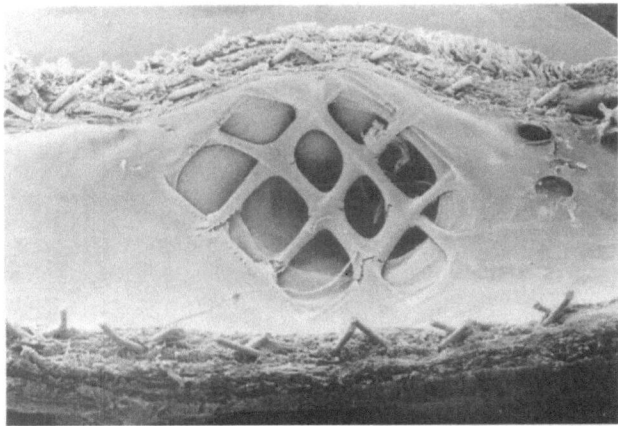

Fig. 2. Electron microscopy of neoendothelium covering a self-expanding stent 9 months after coronary implantation in a dog with a patent side-branch

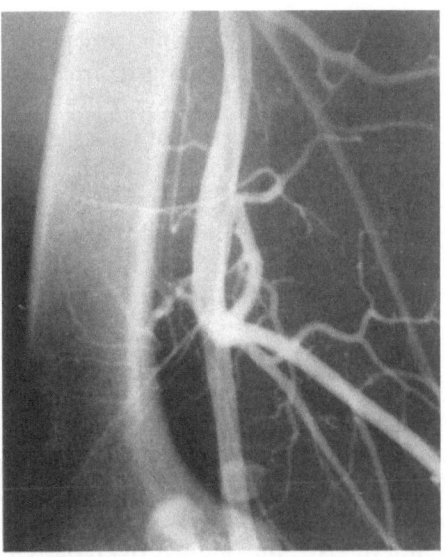

Fig. 3. Radiograph of a stent in a canine femoral artery; a side branch covered by the stent has remained patent

Unfortunately, no satisfactory animal model exists which can reproduce the clinical situation of a diseased human coronary artery. The human artery may react to an indwelling stent quite differently from an animal artery. The deposition of platelets and fibrin almost certainly occurs within the first hours of deployment, but the endothelial covering may be a much more protracted process [16]. In animal models intravascular stents rarely stimulate marked fibrointimal hyperplasia. However, fibrointimal proliferation does occur around stented human vessels perhaps due to the scarring process

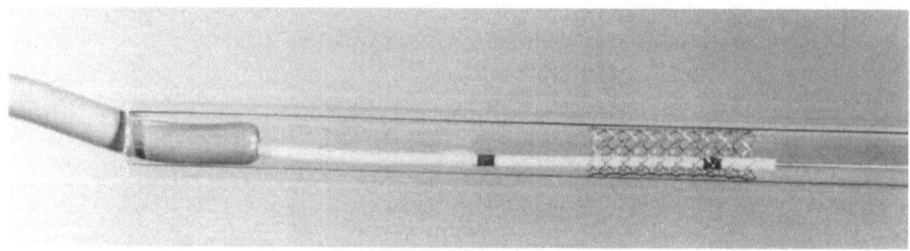

Fig. 4. Introducer and self-expanding stent through an 8 French guiding catheter, over an exchange guidewire (reprinted with permission from [74])

from previous angioplasty procedures [25]. It's clear that new mechanical devices may yield unpredictable results when human studies are performed.

Deployment of the Self-Expanding Mesh Stent

During elective stenting procedures, angioplasty of the target lesion is carried out using standard procedures. The balloon catheter is withdrawn over an exchange guidewire (300 cm) which is positioned across the lesion. The stent is sized such that its unconstrained diameter is 15%–20% larger than the normal diameter of the angioplastied segment. This size differential not only exerts some residual radial force on the vessel wall, but it also insures that the stent will be in contact along the full extent of the wall.

The introducing system is advanced over the guidewire (Fig. 4) with the stent carefully positioned across the previously dilated area. Since the stent contracts along its long axis as its diameter expands, the operator must visually estimate where the fully expanded stent will finally be positioned. Considerable experience usually is required for this maneuver. (This expertise may explain, partially, the different results obtained by various operators around the world.) The constraining membrane is inflated under a pressure of 3 bars and is then withdrawn slowly under fluoroscopic guidance. This action releases the stent into the vascular lumen. A balloon catheter is reintroduced over the guidewire into the stented segment and a final inflation is done to "smooth" any remaining irregularities (sometimes referred to as the "Swiss Kiss") and insure that the stent is embedded into the vessel wall. Several studies have shown that the improved angiographic appearance after stenting correlates with a marked decrease in the translesional gradient [26] and correlates with substantial improvements in the luminal diameter when measured by quantitative angiography [27, 28].

The introducing system can negotiate tortuous segments and deploy stents in distal locations without difficulty because of its flexibility and tapered tip design. Large diameter arteries or vein grafts can be treated with the same 1.57 mm diameter introducing catheter used for small vessels since the expansion ratio of the stent is excellent (3.0–6.5 mm). We have not had problems of stent migration or premature stent release, and embolization has not occurred.

Indications for Coronary Stenting

A) Abrupt Closure. Several risk factors which may lead to abrupt occlusion are now known [29–31], but it remains an unpredictable event. Abrupt occlusion probably arises from major intimal flaps which reduce flow and promote thrombus formation along with the potential for vessel wall recoil [32–34]. The standard management of this complication involves repeated balloon dilatations, often with prolonged, low pressure inflations and the use of a slight increase in balloon size. The angioplasty guidewire often affords some degree of protection against complete occlusion, unless the event happens after its removal. Reperfusion catheters can maintain forward flow while effectively "stenting" the dissection for a brief period of time [35, 36]. Unfortunately, thrombus may form in these catheters while the patient is on the way to surgery for a definitive procedure.

In most series, emergency surgical revascularization is necessary for approximately half the cases of abrupt closure [37]. The operation is associated with an increased morbidity and mortality when compared with elective procedures [38, 39]. The incidence of myocardial infarction varies between 31% and 71% [37, 40] due to the unavoidable delay between vessel occlusion and surgical revascularization, and in-hospital mortality has been reported to be as high as 15% [37]. The risks of abrupt closure and its associated morbidity and mortality limit the patients for whom angioplasty is an acceptable alternative to bypass surgery.

Other approaches to the problem of abrupt closure are under evaluation. The laser balloon has successfully treated this complication, but preliminary reports suggest a significant rate of restenosis [41, 42]. Temporary intravascular stents are intended to tack up an intimal flap and insure normal flow for a brief time period, but thus far they have been used successfully only in a small group of patients [43]. We will discuss the role of the self-expanding mesh stent in abrupt closure later in the chapter.

B) Coronary Artery Restenosis. The mechanism of restenosis is under intense investigation, but our knowledge is still limited. Pathological studies in animals and man have shown that angioplasty involves fissuring of plaque material, sometimes to the level of the internal elastic membrane [33, 44]. The initial plaque disruption and the rheological consequences of a suboptimal balloon dilatation leads to the deposition of platelets and fibrin along the vessel wall. Mitogens are released both by the vessel wall and

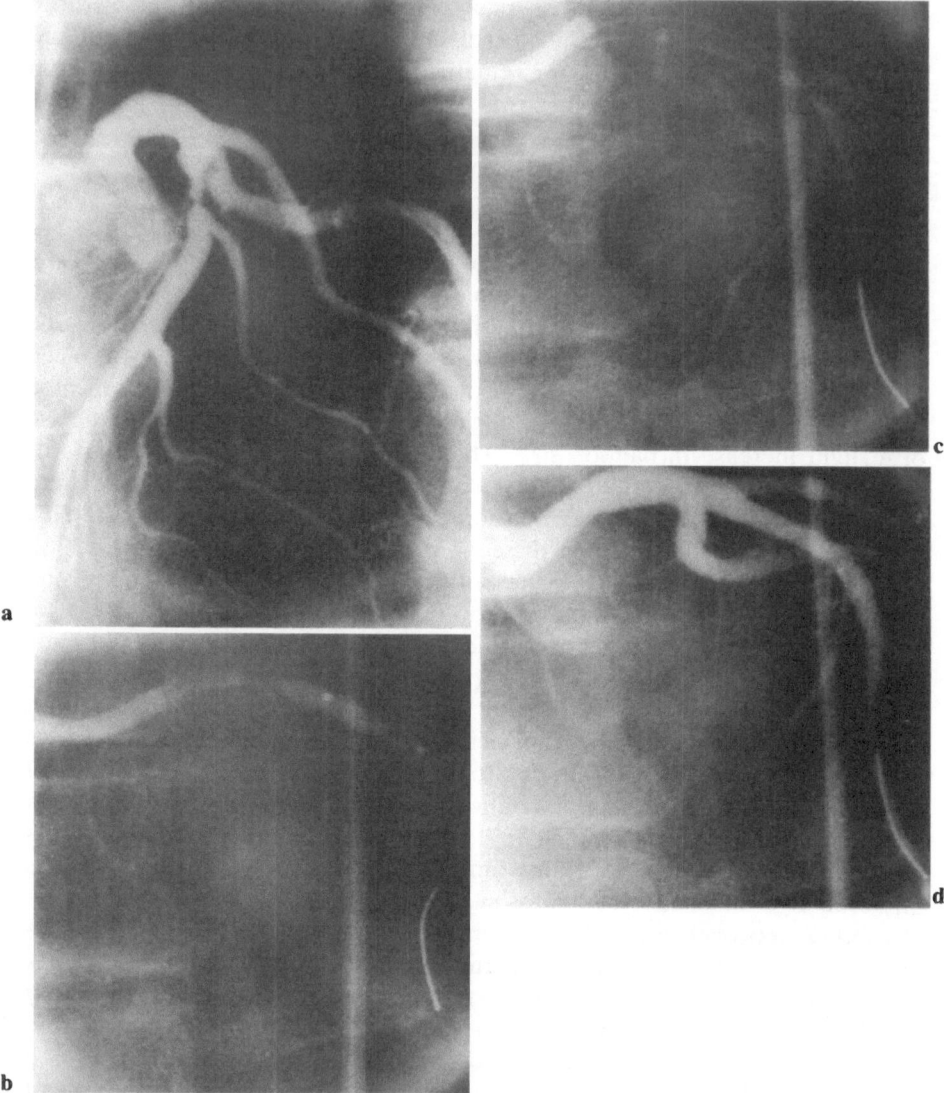

Fig. 5a–d. Elective use of the self-expanding stent for prevention of recurrent restenosis in a 62-year-old patient with NYSHA class III angina 4 months after standard angioplasty. **a** Left anterior oblique, cranial view of a tight restenosis in the left anterior descending coronary artery. **b** Right anterior oblique view of the same vessel showing the guide wire and delivery system for stent implantation. **c** Same view now showing the stent deployed in the vessel; the guide wire is still in place. **d** Right anterior oblique view showing the vessel after successful deployment of the stent with excellent flow and no evidence of residual stenosis. At 1 year follow-up, the patient was asymptomatic and had no angiographic evidence of restenosis

platelets which cause migration of smooth muscle cells to the damaged area [45]. The compromised flow and the amount of intimal and medial damage may be among the early triggers that initiate the fibromuscular proliferation of "late" restenosis [44, 46, 47]. Early restenosis typically occurs in the first 4–6 weeks after the procedure and usually is due to vascular recoil at the site of the original balloon dilatation, coronary spasm, or a major intimal flap limiting flow and which is further compromised by fresh thrombus (Fig. 5).

Standard balloon dilatations with various sized balloons inflated with either low or high pressure inflations, for a short or prolonged duration, have not altered the incidence of these complications [48–50]. Adjunctive medical therapy also has had little effect on rates of restenosis [51]. Investigators, therefore, have turned to mechanical alternatives to balloon angioplasty. Interventionalists have attempted to remove excessive atherosclerotic material instead of dilating the stenotic arterial segment by pulverizing the lesion with mechanical drills [52, 53]. They have melted atheroma with laser energy delivered through an optical fiber or radiofrequency heated elements, both of which are integrated into a balloon catheter [54–56]. Others are attempting to "debulk" atheroma by shaving the plaque with percutaneous atherectomy devices [57].

We have deployed self-expanding mesh stents for coronary artery restenosis and will discuss these results later in the chapter. A stent produces a smooth surface and normal flow and will prevent the elastic recoil from a dilated vascular wall making it a logical device for this problem. However, an intravascular foreign-body theoretically could contribute to smooth muscle cell proliferation. The stent could act as a mechanical irritant causing the release of mediators from the adjacent endothelium stimulating coronary spasm or intimal hyperplasia. Perhaps most worrisome, the device can become a nidus for the development of thrombus.

C) Saphenous Vein Graft Stenosis. Balloon angioplasty within venous bypass grafts is well documented as having a higher restenosis rate than in native coronary arteries. If the lesion is in the body of the graft, restenosis rates as high as 60% have been reported [58]. Stenting grafts appears an attractive alternative to these high restenosis rates. It is especially appealing since repeat coronary artery bypass surgery has a lower likelihood of success and an increased morbidity and mortality when compared to a first operation [59].

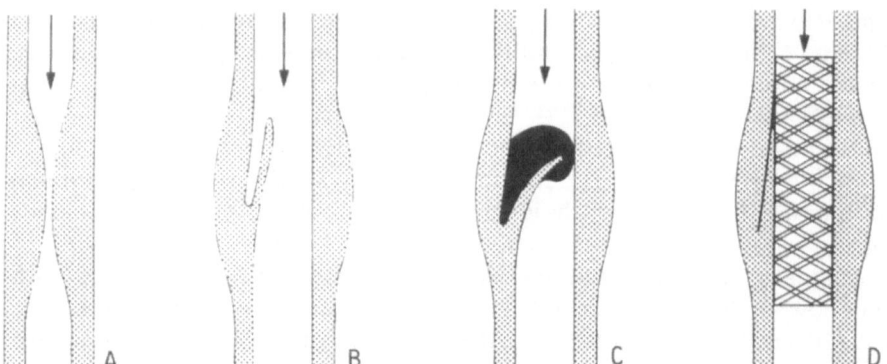

Fig. 6. Diagramatic representation of a self-expanding stent implantation for acute occlusion. *A*, Coronary stenosis before balloon angioplasty. *B*, After balloon inflation stretching of the arterial segment has been induced, together with plaque rupture. *C*, An intimal flap forms with superimposed thrombus, and this acutely occludes the lumen of the vessel. *D*, Stent implantation "tacks down" the flap and prevents elastic recoil of the dilated segment. (Reprinted with permission from [74])

Clinical Studies Utilizing the Self-Expanding Mesh Stent for Abrupt Occlusion

We reported our early experience from Lausanne using the intracoronary stent for situations of abrupt closure [16]. The study comprised 25 patients who were treated by immediate stenting rather than surgery from April 1986 to December 1988 (Figs. 6, 7). This group represented 60% of all patients at the University of Lausanne who needed emergency revascularization after failed angioplasty. In 24 patients the implantation was technically successful with immediate relief from chest pain and correction of electrocardiographic abnormalities. In 3 cases, acute stent thrombosis was documented angiographically or suspected clinically during the hospital stay. One of these patients was recanalized mechanically by balloon angioplasty. Another patient with suspected stent occlusion died (4%) within 24 h from intractable arrhythmias. He had received a stent to his left anterior descending coronary artery for ongoing myocardial infarction complicated by severe hemodynamic instability. The third patient developed a transmural myocardial infarction.

Five patients from this group (20%) suffered a moderate rise in cardiac enzymes (Fig. 8). We assumed that the myocardial necrosis in one patient was due to the placement of a stent in an area of active thrombus with the subsequent loss of a side branch. Another reason for the enzyme rise was probably due to delays between occlusion and stent implantation [60].

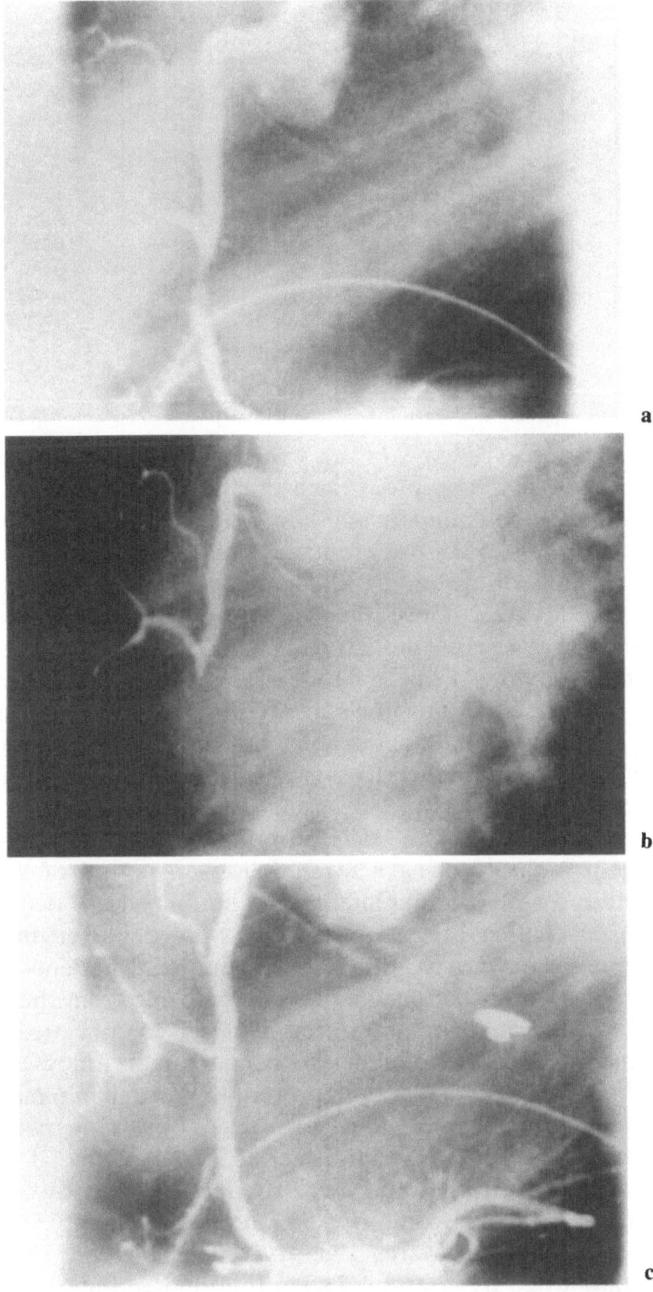

Fig. 7a–c. Self-expanding stent implantation for acute occlusion occuring after balloon coronary angioplasty. **a** Left anteror oblique view of tight mid-lesion in the right coronary artery of 57-year-old patient who presented with severe angina. **b** After balloon angioplasty with a 3.0 mm and then a 3.5 mm balloon, abrupt and irreversible occlusion occurs with severe symptomatic ischemia. **c** After implantation of two stents in tandem, the flow is excellent, and there is no significant residual stenosis. (Reprinted with permission from [16])

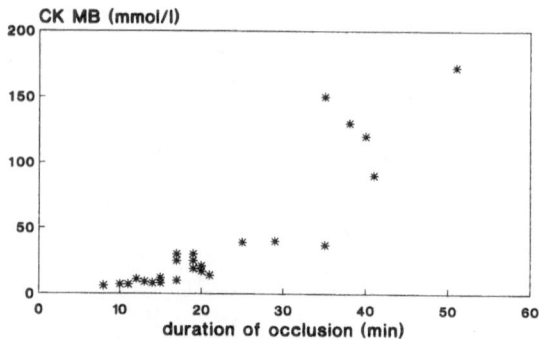

Fig. 8. Analysis of creatine phosphokinase (CPK) results from patients undergoing intra-coronary stenting for abrupt occlusion

In the early days of this experimental procedure we did not have stents available in the hospital. Each situation where a stent was indicated required us to call the company and have a device brought to the cath lab. The time delay led us to the use of intracoronary urokinase in hopes of preventing the formation of thrombus along the guide wire which remained across the occluded area. Once the procedure became more routine, a supply of stents was kept in the lab decreasing the time between occlusion and stent implantation. At that time we stopped using intracoronary urokinase.

The median hospital stay after stent deployment for abrupt closure was 7 days. The initial angiographic follow-up of this patient subgroup suggested that the combined restenosis and late occlusion rate was lower after emergency stenting than after angioplasty alone. The angiographic rate of restenosis was 3/17 (18%) for the patients who underwent late control angiography. During a mean follow-up period of 7 months, two patients suffered a myocardial infarction, and there were two noncardiac deaths.

Since that original report, we have deployed the self-expanding mesh stent for abrupt closure in nine additional patients. One patient required surgical repair because of continued oozing from the femoral puncture site. However, no patient suffered a major complication – Q wave infarction, emergency CABG, or death. Angiographic follow-up is available for four of six patients who had the procedure more than 6 months ago. None of this small group show evidence of restenosis. One patient from Greece has verbally reported no complications.

The European multicenter experience with self-expanding mesh stents for abrupt occlusion comprises 56 patients in whom 63 devices were implanted in 57 sites from March 1986 to December 1989. Eleven cases (20%) were complicated by in-hospital stent thrombosis, but 5 of these were successfully recanalized using balloon angioplasty, thrombolytic treatment, or a combination of both. There were 7 cases of myocardial infarction (13%) and 2 patients died (4%). The approach in the acute setting was not uniform in all centers. Some centers used the stent as a temporary bridge to elective bypass surgery. Seven of the 56 patients underwent surgical revascularization within 24–48 h after the procedure, although they remained clinically stable and myocardial infarction had been prevented. There was considerable variability in the rate of acute stent thrombotic complications between Lausanne (12%) and the other sites (20%). These differences probably reflect differing anticoagulation regimens, patient selection criteria, and an important learning curve effect [61]. At the present time, the data suggest that abrupt occlusion constitutes one of the best indications for coronary stenting.

Clinical Results of the Self-Expanding Stent for Restenosis

Our initial 50 elective stenting procedures of native coronary arteries for restenosis were performed in patients with a mean of 1.6 previous angioplasties at the same site (range 1–4) [17]. In 46 cases, a single stent was deployed, and in 4 cases two or more stents were implanted. All implants were technically successful. Temporary thrombotic occlusion occurred in two cases (4%), and permanent occlusion was observed in two additional cases (4%) during the hospital stay. Two of these patients underwent emergency surgery, one of whom died postoperatively from surgical complications (unrecognized tamponade).

The major complication rate (Q wave infarction, emergency surgery or death) was 6% in-hospital. After a mean follow-up period of 8 months, angiography was repeated in 34 patients from the study group. Restenosis within the stented segment occurred in 4 patients (12%), and stent occlusion was documented in three other patients (9%) [62]. There were three late deaths in the study group (6%). Two of these deaths were probably related to the stent as they occurred in patients who did not adhere to their anticoagulant drug regimen. One death occurred during elective surgery for a new left main stem coronary lesion which occurred proximal to a stent placed near the origin of the left anterior descending artery. Two patients from this group required elective surgery for restenosis within the stent.

Since that report we have stented 22 additional patients for coronary restenosis. No major complications occurred while these patients were hospitalized. Three patients required surgical repair for continued femoral artery bleeding. We have obtained follow-up angiography on 19 patients from this study group. Two patients (10.5%) had evidence of significant stent restenosis defined as greater than 50% luminal narrowing. Thus far, no late complications have occurred in this group of patients.

Several other centers have used the self-expanding mesh stent to treat restenosis. The European experience consists of deploying 118 stents for

112 restenosis lesions in 107 patients from March 1986 to December 1989 (Medinvent, data base). In this series, in-hospital thrombotic complications occurred in 22 cases (20%), five of which were successfully recanalized. Myocardial infarction was observed in 15 patients (14%) and there was one in-hospital death. During follow-up there were 4 cardiac deaths that were possibly related to the implanted stent. The total cardiac mortality for the group was 5%. The differences between the results in Lausanne compared with other centers again probably relates to the patient selection, the type of anticoagulation regimen employed, and the learning curve effect.

. The incidence of restenosis in the multicenter study group is being monitored by a central angiography laboratory at the Thorax Center in Rotterdam. The films are analyzed using the CASS system, a semi-automated, computer-based, method for quantifying coronary luminal diameter [63]. Through March of 1990, 82 patient angiograms were evaluated at least 4 months after stent placement for either restenosis or abrupt closure (Patrick W. Serruys, M.D., personal communication). When restenosis was defined as greater than 50% luminal narrowing, the rate for the stented patients was 6% (5/82) (Fig. 9).

Pending further technical improvements in these devices, the appropriate selection of patients for intracoronary stenting remains central to success, and probably represents the largest portion of the learning curve [61]. The importance of anticoagulants has been repeatedly demonstrated by

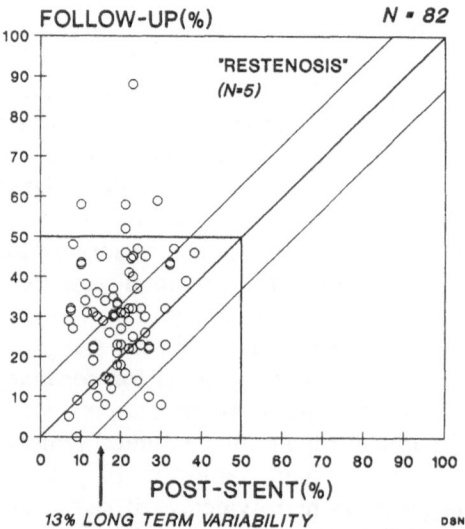

Fig. 9. Multicenter, quantitative, angiographic evaluation of the restenosis rate after implantation of the self-expanding stent in native coronary arteries. Using the 50% diameter stenosis criterium, only 5 patients (6%) in this subgroup have developed restenosis. See text for details. (Courtesy of Patrick W. Serruys, Thoraxcentrum, Erasmus University, Rotterdam)

patients, or their physicians, who discontinued the medication prematurely with disastrous results. In Lausanne we gave each patient a card outlining their anticoagulation medications in three languages, and requesting that any proposed changes be discussed with us before implementation.

Role of the Self-Expanding Mesh Stent in Saphenous Vein Grafts

We have stented 37 patients for stenosis within a saphenous vein bypass graft. (The first 18 patients have been reported previously [18].) On several occasions stenting was done in old grafts that were diffusely diseased and

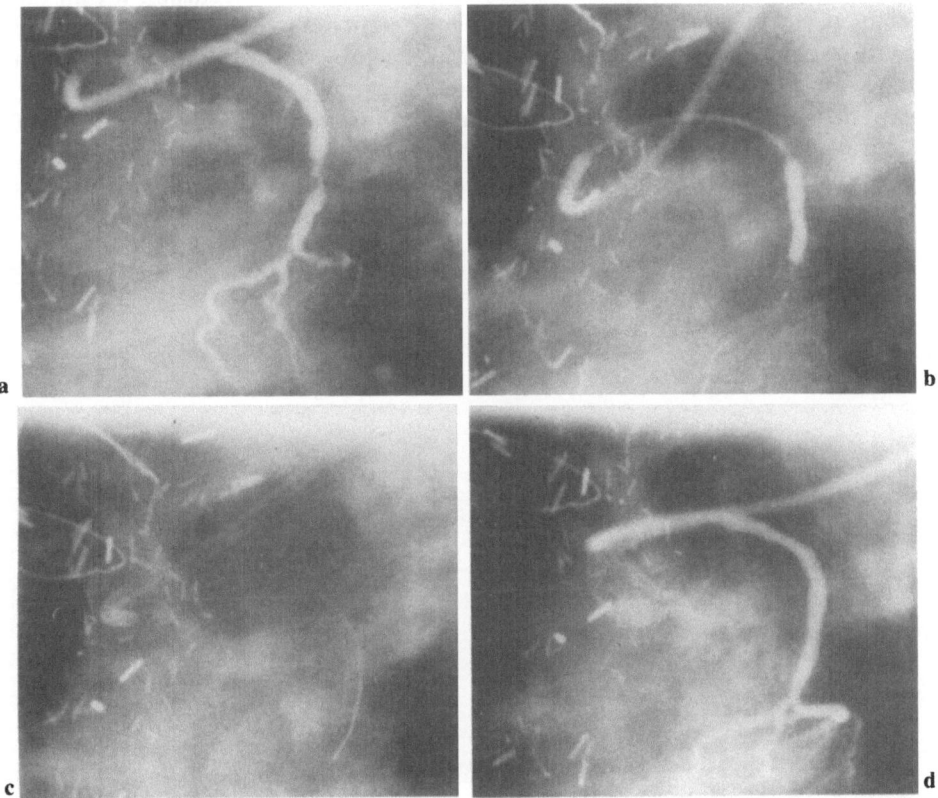

Fig. 10a–d. Self-expanding stent implantation in a saphenous bypass graft. **a** Left anterior oblique view of a well-defined stenosis in the body of a graft to the obtuse marginal branch of the circumflex artery. **b** The self-expanding mesh stent has been placed at the site of the lesion. The guide wire is still present across the stent. **c** After successful stent delivery a balloon is inserted over the guide wire for a single dilatation to help embed the struts into the vessel wall ("Swiss kiss"). **d** After implantation of the stent, no residual stenosis is visible

would not have been considered appropriate targets for balloon angioplasty alone. The implantation procedure for bypass grafts sometimes varied from the one we described for native coronary arteries. To avoid the potential embolization of friable plaque material or thrombus, the stent was inserted before any dilatations were made with a standard balloon catheter.

In this series 27 patients received a single stent (Fig. 10), and 10 patients had two or more stents deployed. There were four cases (11%) of temporary stent thrombosis during the hospital stay. One of these four patients (3%) died suddenly 4 days after the procedure, presumably from an arrhythmia which might have been related to acute stent thrombosis. One patient was recanalized with standard angioplasty and thrombolytic therapy. The third patient had successful bypass surgery, and the last of this group suffered a myocardial infarction. Thirty-three patients have been restudied after a mean follow-up of 9 months. Restenosis, or late occlusion within the stent, occurred in three cases (8%). Three patients (8%) required a second stent implant for a new stenosis outside the previously stented area but in the same bypass graft. There was one death 7 months after implantation in a patient with progressive congestive heart failure who had no suggestion of stent occlusion or restenosis. Another patient died suddenly 3 months after the procedure. Therefore, two late deaths occurred in this group of patients (5%). One patient underwent repeat elective bypass grafting for progression

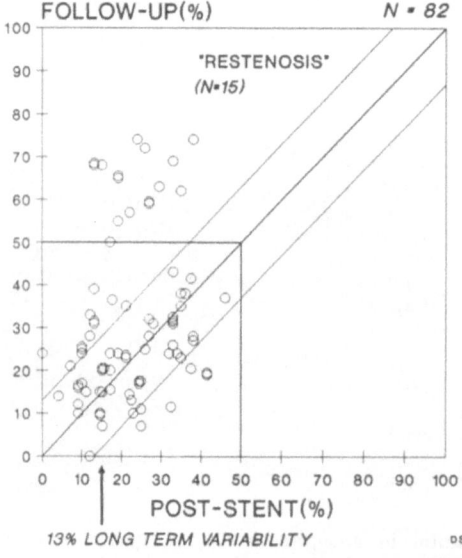

Fig. 11. Multicenter, quantitative, angiographic evaluation of the restenosis rate after implantation of the self-expanding stent in saphenous bypass grafts. Using the 50% diameter stenosis criterium, 15 patients (18%) in this subgroup have developed restenosis. See text for details. (Courtesy of Patrick W. Serruys, Thoraxcentrum, Erasmus University, Rotterdam)

of his disease in other vessels, and the last patient suffered a myocardial infarction after discontinuing her anticoagulants.

The multicenter experience with the self-expanding mesh stent in venous bypass grafts involved the implantation of 146 devices to treat 109 lesions in 76 patients through December 1989 (Medinvent, data base). All procedures were technically successful. Thrombotic complications occurred in 6 cases (8%), one of which was successfully recanalized. There were 6 cases of myocardial infarction (8%) and one in-hospital death. Five other patients died during follow-up, but only one of these deaths occurred from a cardiac cause. Therefore, two deaths are attributable to cardiac causes (3%). Late restenosis in vein grafts is being evaluated by quantitative coronary angiography at the Thoraxcentrum (Fig. 11) [63]. As of March 1990 82 follow-up films (6 months or more after the stenting procedure) have been analyzed. Fifteen patients demonstrated stent occlusion or restenosis (18%), using the criterion of greater than a 50% luminal narrowing defining the presence of a recurrent lesion (Patrick W. Serruys, M.D., personal communication).

The immediate and long-term results for elective stenting of venous bypass grafts with the self-expanding device are better than the results of stenting native coronary vessels. Probably this is due to the larger diameter of vein grafts which allows larger stents to be implanted. Perhaps the lack of vasomotor tone and generally higher compliance of venous bypass grafts also play a role. The combination of an acceptably low complication rate and the low rate of restenosis makes elective stenting of venous bypass grafts the best indication for the use of these devices at this time.

Contraindications for Coronary Stenting

We have developed a list of contraindications to coronary stenting which should be observed whenever possible:

- Lesions situated less than 10 mm from the left main coronary artery
- Markedly funnel-shaped segments (currently available stents are cylindrical)
- Very tight bend in the target segment (since it would promote important shearing forces at both stent extremities)
- Insufficient flow anticipated through the prosthesis after implantation due to either poor distal runoff or extensive collateralization (stasis at stent level will favor thrombus formation)
- Known and documented tendency towards coronary spasm.
- Any anticipated difficulty with the antiplatelet and anticoagulation regimen should constitute an absolute contraindication to stenting with the currently available devices.

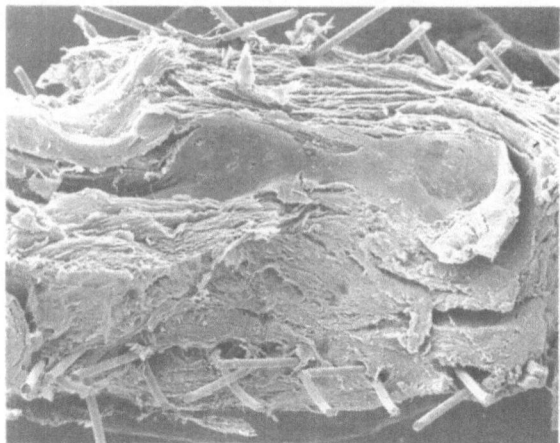

Fig. 12. Severe restenosis within a proximal left anterior descending coronary artery stent that was explanted at the time of elective coronary surgery (reprinted with permission from [64])

Restenosis After Stenting

Experimental animal data, histology from percutaneous atherectomy [57], and surgical material excised from stented segments [64] all suggest that stent restenosis is due to excessive fibrointimal proliferation (Fig. 12). One predictor for stent restenosis appears to be the timing of the deployment after the original angioplasty procedure. In a group of patients treated for restenosis in Lausanne, the recurrence rate was 6% in patients that were stented more than 3 months after their initial angioplasty, but it was 41% for those stented within 3 months. Similar observations have been made with other stents and other devices such as percutaneous directional atherectomy [65]. These findings coupled with the well-known time course for restenosis after standard balloon dilatations suggest that the process of fibrointimal proliferation may have a period of hyperactivity which will be difficult to alter with mechanical interventions alone.

Investigators have also observed the development of excessive hyper-plasia at the self-expanding stent extremities in several cases [18]. This process is probably similar to the "hump" of fibromuscular proliferation sometimes seen at the extremities of these devices in animal studies. In theory, this could be caused by mechanical strain, by progression of native disease, or by a segment dilated by the angioplasty balloon but not covered by the stent. This type of lesion has usually been amenable to further stenting when it was considered clinically significant. The problem has largely disappeared with the use of longer stents that can cover the entire length involved in an angioplasty. Early in our experience, however, one such case did undergo surgery when a tight stenosis developed at the distal extremity of a stent 5 months after its implantation for a left anterior descending lesion. The distal end of the stent was implanted into an intra-myocardial arterial segment with marked extrinsic compression ("milking") during systole. The localized mechanical strain at the stent edge presumably caused the excessive fibromuscular proliferation (Dr. Anthony F. Rickards, personal communication).

Spasm has been observed at the stent extremities immediately after implantation, but has always been transient and responded to intracoronary administration of a vasodilator (e.g., nifedipine). Theoretically, it is possible that intravascular stents may induce spasm over longer periods of time. Spasm could lead to major complications including low flow and thrombotic occlusion of the stented segment.

Treatment of Stent Restenosis

Late fibromuscular restenosis in the area covered by a stent has been amenable to repeat balloon angioplasty, but the improvement has mostly been short-lived [64]. Percutaneous directional atherectomy has been successfully used in one case as a palliative measure, but the stenosis re-curred once again [64]. Coronary stenting does not jeopardize the patient's chances of benefiting from elective surgical revascularization should it become necessary [64].

Complications of Intracoronary Stenting

The process of inserting the self-expanding mesh stent normally is not a source of complications. The stent deployment only adds a few minutes to the procedure's time. Removing the retaining membrane which holds the self-expanding stent on the introducer catheter occasionally can be difficult. In most situations this problem responds to increasing the pressure beyond 3 bars between the membranes, but rarely the position of the guide catheter also must be changed before the membrane can be fully withdrawn. Partially deployed stents have been removed without important sequel. Investigators have not seen evidence of side branch occlusion except in the case where a stent was placed in an area of fresh thrombus that involved a side branch. There have been no cases of coronary perforation, stent erosion, or infectious complications.

The major morbidity associated with stent implantation is the potential for a thrombotic event occurring acutely or, unpredictably, in the first 4 weeks (or even longer) after the procedure. This is in contradistinction to balloon angioplasty where complications generally are not seen beyond the first 24 h after the procedure. A short-term combined anticoagulant and antiplatelet regimen is mandatory. Unfortunately, this leads to local bleeding complications at the arterial puncture site (8% of cases in Lansanne). These patients may require blood transfusions, and some will require surgical repair of the femoral artery before bleeding problems can be controlled. Optimal femoral compression after the procedure is crucial. A pneumatic compression device which allows prolonged pressure without compromising arterial flow is now being tested. Hopefully, this device will help overcome arterial bleeding problems.

Several risk factors for acute stent thrombosis have become apparent. Small diameter stents carry a greater risk of thrombosis than do large ones [62]. This observation probably explains the lower complication rate observed when vein grafts are stented. Generally bypass grafts are at least 3.5 mm in diameter and allow placement of stents at least 4 mm in their unconstrained diameter. We do not recommend stenting arteries that are treated with angioplasty balloons smaller than 3.0 mm with the present generation of devices.

Certain clinical situations promote thrombotic complications. Investigators have noted that patients with increased platelet counts are more likely to experience thrombotic complications [66]. Systemic hypotension, poor distal runoff, untreated significant proximal lesions, and well-developed collaterals can cause decreased flow through the stented vessel and therefore potentiate thrombus formation.

With increasing experience and better patient selection, acute thrombotic events have become less frequent. During the first half of the Lausanne series we observed thrombotic events in 14% of the procedures versus 6% for the last 49 cases [61]. A similar trend has been noted for the multicenter evaluation of the self-expanding stent. Thrombotic complications have decreased from 35% for 1986 ($n = 37$) to 7.5% in 1989 ($n = 80$) (Medinvent data base). Provided a catheterization laboratory is immediately available, acute stent thrombosis can often be treated effectively by balloon angioplasty and thrombolytic agents. When it is reversed, it does not appear to compromise the long-term results [61]. The procedure is fairly straightforward if thrombosis occurs during the first hours after implantation when the femoral sheath is still in place. The situation is more complex after the sheath has been removed because a second arterial puncture becomes necessary in a patient who is anticoagulated. If a thrombotic event occurs more than 3 days after stent deployment, systemic thrombolysis can be beneficial in our experience.

In animal studies a diameter mismatch (ratio >1.5) between the self-expanding stent and the recipient vessel was associated with thrombotic occlusion. Although this degree of mismatch has not been seen in clinical practice, the turbulent flow induced at the stent's extremities could contribute to thrombus formation. This makes optimal sizing an important factor, especially since good impaction of the stent struts into the vessel wall is probably equally important for preventing thrombus formation.

Adjunct Medication

Early experimental evidence showed that heparin significantly decreased the rate of acute thrombotic occlusions when it was given perioperatively for stenting of normal canine arteries [15]. Other workers using balloon-expandable stents in animals showed that aspirin was superior to warfarin in preventing subsequent stent thrombosis [20]. There is some evidence favoring the use of low molecular weight dextran during the implantation procedure together with aspirin, dipyidamole, and heparin [21].

The drug regimen we currently employ with the self-expanding stent largely is empirical. It has been modified recently but still requires a high degree of patient compliance. Before the stent procedure, patients receive aspirin in addition to their usual medication. In the catheterization laboratory, intravenous heparin is administered together with 500–1000 ml of intravenous dextran-40. After the procedure is completed, heparin is continued until oral anticoagulation is effective (International Normalized Ratio for prothrombin time ≥ 2.3). Aspirin 100 mg daily and dipyridamole 100 mg three times daily are prescribed for all patients. Medications are usually continued for 3–6 months, until control angiography is performed. All patients receive calcium blocking agents to prevent the possibility of stent-induced coronary spasm.

Conclusions

The concept of peripheral vascular stenting was introduced over 20 years ago. Major interest in these devices was rekindled when the limitations of coronary balloon angioplasty resisted conventional therapy. Now, after 4 years of clinical study, coronary stenting has given us some reason for optimism. The procedure has lived up to our initial expectations in terms of its technical feasibility. Stents can be inserted under circumstances of abrupt closure and in almost all coronary segments. It is simple to implement and constitutes the best current alternative to emergency surgery for abrupt postangioplasty closure. The data suggests that restenosis may be favorably influenced by stent implantation in selected subgroups, particularly for patients with saphenous vein graft lesions. The "Achilles heel" of coronary stenting remains the problem of acute or subacute thrombosis. Although its incidence appears to be decreasing as our learning curve progresses, it makes a complex drug regimen mandatory increasing the risks of the procedure. Late stent restenosis rates are encouraging, but the data is confounded by the early rates of thrombotic complications. It's unclear what effect might be achieved on late restenosis rates if the high rates of early thrombotic complications could be avoided, or substantially decreased. Moreover, the potential for thrombotic complications and restenosis limits the applicability of stents.

We believe that coronary stents are one of the most promising developments in the field of interventional cardiology. The devices are rapidly evolving and will require more study before they will be ready for general clinical use. It would be interesting to compare these devices to standard angioplasty. However, it took balloon angioplasty over 13 years to develop sufficiently before direct randomized comparisons with surgery and medical treatment seemed appropriate [67]. A similar pattern will probably have to be followed for coronary stents and other new interventional techniques in order to derive meaningful conclusions.

Many researchers in the field of interventional cardiology now believe that the fight against restenosis will have to include the use of pharmacological weapons, not only mechanical means [68, 69]. Whether a combination of these two approaches will finally prove optimal is an unresolved issue. It seems likely that new devices will be forthcoming which will be less thrombogenic and less likely to stimulate intimal hyperplasia.

Radiopaque stents are now entering clinical study which should make the deployment easier and more precise. Other, more complex, innovations are also on the horizon. Muhlestein et al. from Duke University have described the use of a tantalum, single-wire stent, that was implanted percutaneously in peripheral arteries of dogs [70]. After implantation and complete release, it could be straightened and retrieved percutaneously using a modified bioptome catheter. Temporary stents could theoretically obviate the need for long term anticoagulation. Another temporary stent, a basketlike device developed by Gaspard et al., has been used successfully in a small group of patients [45]. More temporary devices for abrupt occlusion will shortly enter clinical evaluation.

Bioresorbable polymers are being examined in vitro with the hope that a temporary nonmetallic support may also decrease thrombus formation and alleviate the need for anticoagulant therapy [71]. A few of these devices have been studied in animal models. Two chapters in this book are devoted to this promising development.

Two groups have demonstrated that seeding of metallic stents with endothelial cells is feasible in vitro, and these stents can be implanted successfully in the experimental animal [72]. Dichek et al. from the National Institute of Health have taken the cellular seeding concept one step further and reported the use of genetically engineered cells which are attached to the stent prior to implantation and markedly enhance the local secretion of t-PA [73]. This elegant intervention is one of the ways drugs may be delivered locally to the stent "environment". The seeded stent may represent a better means of insuring antithrombotic protection while avoiding the complications of systemic anticoagulants. Unfortunately, we don't know how important platelet deposition is to the development of endotheliazation. If these new antithrombotic devices delay or prevent this process, late complications may loom as a major issue. The amount of ongoing stent research demonstrates the importance so many investigators attach to this experimental technique. It also supports our optimism that modifications in the present first generation devices will lead to solutions which will overcome the dual angioplasty problems of abrupt closure and restenosis.

References

1. Dotter CT, Judkins MP (1964) Transluminal treatment of atherosclerotic obstruction: description of a new techdnique and preliminary report of its application. Circulation 30:654–660
2. Gruntzig A (1978) Transluminal dilatation of coronary artery stenoses. Lancet 1:263
3. De Feyter PJ, Serruys PW, van den Brand M et al. (1985) Emergency coronary angioplasty in refractory unstable angina. N Engl J Med 313:342–346
4. Detre K, Holubkov PH, Kelsey S et al. (1988) Percutaneous transluminal coronary angioplasty in 1985–1986 and 1977–1981. N Engl J Med 318:265–270
5. Myler RK, Topol EJ, Shaw RE et al. (1987) Multiple vessel coronary angioplasty: classification, results, and patterns of restenosis in 494 consecutive patients. Cathet Cardiovasc Diagn 13:1–15
6. Traisnel G, Lablanche JM, Fournier JL et al. (1986) Etude comparative des résultats à court et moyen terme de l'angioplastie et du pontage dans l'angor sévère ou instable par sténose isolée de l'IVA. Arch Mal Coeur 10:1430–1436
7. Reeder GS, Krishan I, Nobrega FT et al. (1984) Is percutaneous transluminal coronary angioplasty less expensive than bypass surgery? N Engl J Med 311:1157–1162
8. Laird-Meeter K, Erdman RAM, van Domburg R et al. (1989) Probability of return to work after either coronary balloon dilatation or coronary bypass surgery. Eur Heart J 10:917–922
9. Kramer JR, Proudfit WL, Loop FD et al. (1989) Late follow-up of 781 patients undergoing percutaneous transluminal coronary angioplasty or coronary artery bypass grafting for an isolated obstruction in the left anterior descending coronary artery. Am Heart J 118:1144–1153
10. Ellis SG, Roubin GS, King SB et al. (1988) In-hospital cardiac mortality after coronary angioplasty: analysis of risk factors from 8207 procedures. J Am Coll Cardiol 11:211–216
11. Leimgruber PP, Roubin GS, Hollman J et al. (1986) Restenosis after successful coronary angioplasty in patients with single-vessel disease. Circulation 73:710–717
12. Meier B (1988) Restenosis after coronary angioplasty: review of the literature. Eur Heart J 9 [Suppl C]:1–6
13. Anderson HV, Roubin GS, Leimgruber PP, Douglas JS et al. (1985) Primary angiographic success rates of percutaneous transluminal coronary angioplasty. Am J Cardiol 56:712–716
14. Urban P, Meier B, Finci L et al. (1987) Coronary wedge pressure: a predictor of restenosis after angioplasty. J Am Coll Cardiol 10:504–509
15. Sigwart U, Puel J, Mirkovitch V, Joffre F, Kappenberger L (1987) Intravascular stents to prevent occlusion and restenosis after transluminal angioplasty. N Engl J Med 316:701–706

16. Sigwart U, Urban P, Golf S et al. (1988) Emergency stenting for acute occlusion following coronary balloon angioplasty. Circulation 78:1121–1127
17. Sigwart U, Kaufmann U, Goy JJ et al. (1988) Prevention of coronary restenosis by stenting. Eur Heart J 9 [Suppl C]:31–37
18. Urban P, Sigwart U, Golf S et al. (1989) Intravascular stenting for stenosis of aorto-coronary venous bypass grafts. J Am Coll Cardiol 13:1085–1091
19. Rousseau H, Puel J, Joffre F, Sigwart U et al. (1987) Self-expanding endovascular prosthesis: an experimental study. Radiology 164:709–714
20. Roubin GS, Robinson KA, King SB et al. (1987) Early and late results of intracoronary arterial stenting after coronary angioplasty in dogs. Circulation 76:891–897
21. Palmaz JC, Garcia OJ, Kopp DT et al. (1987) Balloon expandable intra-arterial stents: effect of anticoagulation on thrombus formation (abstract). Circulation 76 [Suppl IV]:IV-45
22. Schatz RA, Palmaz JC, Tio FO et al. (1987) Balloon-expandable intracoronary stents in the adult dog. Circulation 76:450–457
23. Palmaz JC, Sibbitt RR, Tio FO et al. (1986) Expandable intraluminal vascular graft: a feasibility study. Surgery 99:199–205
24. Palmaz JC (1988) Balloon-expandable intravascular stents. Am J Radiol 150:1263–1269
25. Urban P, Sigwart U, Kaufmann U, Kappenberger L (1989) Restenosis within coronary stents: possible effect of previous angioplasty (abstract). J Am Coll Cardiol 13:107A
26. Sigwart U, Kaufmann U, Goy JJ, Kappenberger L (1987) Suppression of residual transstenotic pressure gradient after PTCA by implantation of self expanding stents (abstract). Circulation 76 [Suppl IV]:IV-186
27. Puel J, Juillière Y, Bertrand M, Rickards A et al. (1988) Early and late assessment in stenosis geometry after coronary arterial stenting. Am J Cardiol 61:546–553
28. Serruys PW, Juillière Y, Bertrand M et al. (1988) Additional improvement of stenosis geometry in human coronary arteries by stenting after balloon dilatation. Am J Cardiol 61:71G–76G
29. Simpfendorfer C, Belardi J, Bellamy G et al. (1987) Frequency, management and follow-up of patients with acute coronary occlusions after percutaneous transluminal coronary angioplasty. Am J Cardiol 59:267–269
30. Mabin TA, Holmes DR, Smith HC et al. (1985) Intracoronary thrombus: role in coronary occlusion complicating percutaneous transluminal coronary angioplasty. J Am Coll Cardiol 5:198–202
31. Roubin GS, Douglas JS, King SB et al. (1988) Influence of balloon size on initial success, acute complications and restenosis after percutaneous transluminal coronary angioplasty. A randomized study. Circulation 78:557–565
32. Waller BF (1989) Crackers, breakers, stretchers, shavers, burners, welders and melters. The future treatment of atherosclerotic coronary artery disease? A clinical and morphological assessment. J Am Coll Cardiol 13:969–987
33. Cragg A, Amplatz K (1986) Vascular pathophysiology of transluminal angioplasty. In: Jang GD (ed) Angioplasty. McGraw-Hill, New York, pp 145–155
34. Block PC (1984) Mechanism of transluminal angioplasty. Am J Cardiol 53:69C–78C
35. Quigley PJ, Hinohara T, Philips HR et al. (1988) Myocardial protection during coronary balloon angioplasty with an autoperfusion balloon catheter in humans. Circulation 78:1128–1134
36. Hinohara T, Simpson JB, Phillips HR, Stack RS (1988) Transluminal intracoronary reperfusion catheter: a device to maintain coronary perfusion between failed coronary angioplasty and emergency coronary bypass surgery. J Am Coll Cardiol 11:977–982
37. Meier B (1988) Coronary angioplasty. Grune and Stratton, Orlando
38. Page US, Okies JE, Colburn LQ et al (1986) Percutaneous transluminal coronary angioplasty. A growing surgical problem. J Thorac Cardiovasc Surg 92:847–852

39. Satter P, Krause E, Skupin M Mortality trends in cases of elective and emergency aorto-coronary bypass after percutaneous transluminal angioplasty. Thorac Cardiovasc Surg 35:2–5
40. Reul GJ, Cooley DA, Hallman GL et al. (1984) Coronary artery bypass for unsuccessful percutaneous transluminal coronary angioplasty. J Thorac Cardiovasc Surg 88:685–690
41. Spears JR, Reyes VP, Sinclair N et al. (1989) Percutaneous coronary laser balloon angioplasty: preliminary results of a multicenter trial (abstract). J Am Coll Cardiol 13:61A
42. Spears JR, Reyes VP, Plokker HWT et al. (1990) Laser balloon angioplasty: coronary angiographic follow-up of a multicenter trial (abstract). J Am Coll Cardiol 15:26A
43. Gaspard PE, Didier BP, Delsanti GL (1990) The temporary stent catheter: a non operative treatment for acute occlusion during coronary angioplasty (abstract). J Am Coll Cardiol 15:118A
44. Liu MW, Roubin GS, King SB (1989) Restenosis after coronary angioplasty. Potential biologic determinants and role of intimal hyperplasia. Circulation 79:1374–1387
45. Steele PM, Chesebro JH, Stanson AW et al. (1985) Balloon angioplasty: natural history of the pathophysiological response to injury in a pig model. Circ Res 57:105–112
46. Reidy MA, Silver M (1985) Endothelial regeneration VII. Lack of intimal proliferation after defined injury to rat aorta. Am J Pathol 118:173–177
47. Lyon RT, Zarens CK, Lu CJ et al. (1987) Vessel, plaque, and human morphology after transluminal balloon angioplasty: quantitative study in distended human arteries. Arterio sclerosis 7:306–314
48. Roubin GS, Douglas TJ, King SB et al. (1988) Influence of balloon size on initial success, acute complications, and restensosis after percutaneous transluminal coronary angiopalsty: a prospective randomized study. Circulation 78:557–565
49. Meier B, Gruentzig A, King SB et al. (1984) Higher balloon dilatation pressure in coronary angioplasty. Am Heart J 107:619–622
50. Garrahy PJ, Nath H, Anderson JC et al. (1989) Does balloon inflation duration influence the angiographic result in coronary angioplasty (abstract)? J Am Coll Cardiol 13:58A
51. Blackshew JL, O'Callaghan WG, Califf RM (1987) Medical approaches to the prevention of restenosis after coronary angioplasty. J Am Coll Cardiol 9:834–848
52. Hansen DD, Auth DC, Hall M, Ritchie JL (1988) Rotational endarterectomy in normal canine coronary arteries: preliminary report. J Am Coll Cardiol 11:1073–1077
53. Vallbracht C, Liermann D, Prignitz I et al. (1988) Results of low speed rotational angioplasty for chronic total occlusions. Am J Cardiol 62:935–940
54. Abela GS, Seeger JM, Barbieri E et al. (1986) Laser angioplasty with angioscopic guidance in humans. J Am Coll Cardiol 8:184–192
55. Crea F, Davies G, McKenna WJ et al. (1988) Laser recanalisation of coronary arteries by metal-capped optical fibres: early clinical experience in patients with stable angina pectoris. Br Heart J 59:168–174
56. Karsch KR, Haase KK, Voelker W et al. (1990) Percutaneous coronary excimer laser angioplasty in patients with stable and unstable angina pectoris. Circulation 81:1849–1859
57. Simpson JB, Rowe M, Robertson G et al. (1990) Directional coronary atherectomy: success and complication rates and outcome predictors (abstract). J Am Coll Cardiol 15:196A
58. Côté G, Myler RK, Stertzer SH et al. (1987) Percutaneous transluminal angioplasty of stenotic coronary artery grafts: 5 years' experience. J Am Coll Cardiol 9:8–17
59. Loop FD, Cosgrove DM, Kramer JR (1981) Late clinical and arteriographic results in 500 coronary artery reoperations. J Thorac Cardiovasc Surg 81:675–685

60. Sigwart U, Vogt P, Goy JJ, Urban P et al. (1989) Creatinine Kinase levels after bail-out stenting for post angioplasty coronary occlusion (abstract). Circulation 80:II-258
61. Sigwart U, Urban P, Sadeghi H, Kappenberger L (1989) Implantation of 100 intracoronary stents. Learning curve effect on the occurrence of acute complications (abstract). J Am Coll Cardiol 13:107A
62. Sigwart U, Golf S, Kaufmann U, Kappenberger L (1988) Analysis of complications associated with coronary stenting (abstract). J Am Coll Cardiol 11:66A
63. Serruys PW, Reiber JH, Wijns W et al. (1984) Assessment of percutaneous transluminal coronary angioplasty by quantitative coronary angiography: diameter versus densitometric area measurements. Am J Cardiol 54:482–488
64. Sigwart U, Kaufmann U, Golf S, Urban P et al. (1988) L'incidence et le traitement de la resténose coronarienne malgré l'implantation d'une endoprothèse. Schweiz Med Wochenschr 118:1715–1718
65. Selmon M, Robertson G, Hinohara T et al. (1989) Factors associated with restenosis following successful peripheral atherectomy (abstract). J Am Coll Cardiol 13:13A
66. Leon MB, Almagor Y, Erbel R et al. (1989) Subacute thrombotic events after coronary stent placement: clinical spectrum and predictive factors (abstract). Circulation 80:II-174
67. Henderson RA (1989) The randomised Intervention treatment of angina (RITA) trial protocol: a long term study of coronary angioplasty and coronary bypass surgery in patients with angina. Br Heart J 62:411–414
68. Serruys PW, Beatt KJ, van der Giessen WJ (1989) Stenting of coronary arteries. Are we the sorcerer's apprentice? Eur Heart J 10:774–782
69. King SB (1989) Vascular stents and atherosclerosis. Circulation 79:460–462
70. Muhlestein JB, Quigley PJ, Mikat EM et al. (1989) Percutaneous removal of endovascular stents: initial experimental results (abstract). Circulation 80:II-259
71. Slepian MJ, Schindler A (1988) Polymeric endoluminal paving/sealing: a biodegradable alternative to intracoronary stenting (abstract). Circulation 78 [Suppl II]:II-409
72. Van der Giessen WJ, Serruys PW, Visser WJ et al. (1988) Endothelialization of intravascular stents. J Interven Cardiol 1:109–120
73. Dichek DA, Neville RF, Zweibel JA et al. (1989) Seeding of intravascular stents with genetically engineered endothelial cells. Circulation 80:1347–1353
74. Sigwart U, Urban P (1989) Use of coronary stents following balloon angioplasty. In: Braunwald E (ed) Heart disease – update, vol 5. Saunders, Philadelphia, p 111

Report of the Initial Experience with the Palmaz-Schatz Coronary Stent Following Elective Angioplasty

R.A. Schatz,[1] P.S. Teirstein,[1] J. Hirshfeld[2], H. Cabin,[3] M. Savage,[4] and M. Buchbinder[5]

Introduction

Vascular stents have been proposed by multiple investigators as potential solutions to abrupt closure and restenosis following PTCA in man [1, 2]. Direct comparison of the various stent designs with regard to safety and efficacy is not possible due to the absence of side by side controlled studies. Since the techniques required to deliver these devices are rapidly evolving, such comparisons would be premature. The largest experience worldwide thus far has been with the Palmaz–Schatz coronary stent developed by Johnson & Johnson Interventional Systems (Warren, New Jersey) and thus will be the subject of this chapter.

Background

Figure 1 illustrates the first balloon expandable stent to reach clinical trials in humans. This segmented tubular stent is made of stainless steel and measures 1.5 mm in diameter by 15 mm in length. The walls are etched into multiple rows of staggered rectangles that allow for balloon expansion to a maximum diameter of 5–6 mm. This design represents a modification of Palmaz's original rigid stent design used successfully in a large series of patients with iliac artery stenosis [3].

Entry Criteria

Patients were enrolled prospectively into this study based upon the following criteria: (1) greater than 70% narrowing of a major native coronary artery

[1] Cardiology Division of the Scripps Clinic and Research Foundation, La Jolla, CA, [2] University of Pennsylvania Medical Center, [3] Yale Hospital, New Haven, CT, [4] Thomas Jefferson University Hospital, Philadelphia, PA, [5] University of California, San Diego, CA, USA
Address for Correspondence: R.A. Schatz, Arizona Heart Institute Foundation, 4800 North, 22th Street, PO Box 100000, Phoenix, AZ 85064, USA

Coronary Stents
Edited by U. Sigwart and G.I. Frank
© Springer-Verlag Berlin Heidelberg 1992

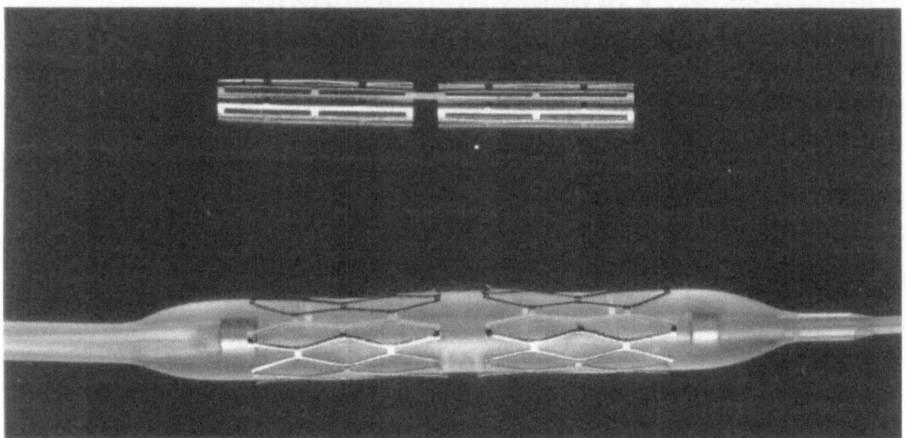

Fig. 1. The Palmaz–Schatz coronary stent (Johnson & Johnson Interventional Systems, Warren, NJ)

($\geqslant 2.5$ mm in diameter, but $\leqslant 5$ mm in diameter); (2) lesion length $\leqslant$ to 15 mm (single stent); (3) symptoms of angina pectoris despite medical therapy or an abnormal thallium stress test in the distribution of the target vessel; (4) ability to give informed consent; (5) the patient otherwise is a good surgical candidate. Patients were excluded if the target vessel was extremely tortuous, the lesion very distal, or if there was poor runoff. Lesions of saphenous vein bypass grafts were also eliminated as were patients suffering from abrupt closure following routine angioplasty or if they had suffered a recent myocardial infarction. Stenting of the left main coronary artery was considered a contraindication unless protected by one or more saphenous vein bypass grafts.

Methods

The patients were treated with calcium channel blockers, aspirin and dipyridamole for 24–48 h prior to and for 3 months after stenting. Low molecular weight dextran 40 was given intravenously at 100 cc/h for 2 h prior to stenting, then at 50–100 cc/h until 1 liter was infused. Ten thousand units of heparin was given during the procedure followed by additional doses to maintain the activated clotting time at 300 s. After an initial pilot study (39 patients) all patients in the series were treated with warfarin for 1–3 months post procedure [4]. All films were sent to a central core lab for quantitative analysis.

Results

A total of 247 patients was enrolled in the study prospectively, 192 of whom were male, 55 were female. The average age of the patients was 58 years (range 27–86). Some 70% of the patients had previous angioplasty which had resulted in restenosis. The distribution of vessels stented were right coronary artery 134, left anterior descending (LAD) 78, circumflex/obtuse marginal branch 31, left main 4. In all, 198 patients received single stents, and 49 received anywhere from 2–6 multiple stents in tandem.

Stent delivery was successful in 94% of the patients attempted. The outcome of those patients in whom failed delivery occurred has been reported previously [5]. Delivery success has improved to greater than 99% with the introduction of a 5F subselective sheath (Teleguide, Schneider, Minneapolis, MN). This device prevents stent-wall contact until deployment of the stent and thus eliminates snagging and embolization, both previously reported as complications in a small percentage of patients [4]. The focus of this paper will be the clinical outcome of those patients in whom stent delivery was successful. Furthermore, a pilot study without anticoagulation in 39 patients has also been previously reported and has been excluded from this analysis [5].

Table 1 describes the complications that have occurred in the 247 patients in whom stent delivery was successful and who were anticoagulated. Acute closure described as total stent thrombosis within 24 h of stent delivery did not occur. Subacute thrombosis defined as total stent thrombosis between 24 h and 2 weeks occurred in 7 (2.8%) patients. Of these 7 patients, one developed a Q wave myocardial infarction, and 2 developed non-Q wave myocardial infarction. Four were sent to urgent bypass surgery for guiding catheter or wire dissection ($n = 3$) or subacute closure ($n = 1$). There were no deaths related to stent thrombosis, but there was one cerebrovascular accident 2 months post procedure, one sudden death at 4 months in a patient with a normal stress test and no angina, and 1 malignancy-related death at 2 years.

Major bleeding complications requiring either transfusion or surgical repair occurred in 24 (9.7%) patients. Therefore a major complication such

Table 1. Complications following coronary stenting ($n = 247$ patients)

Acute closure (<24 h)	0
Subacute closure (>24 h)	7 (2.8%)
Myocardial infarct	3 (1.2%)
Death, stent thrombosis	0
Death, other	3 (1.2%)
Urgent CABG	4 (1.6%)
Bleeding	24 (9.7%)

Table 2. Quantitative analysis of annual angiography following coronary stenting ($n = 33$ lesions/31 patients)

	Pre	Post	6 months	12 months
Minimal lumen diameter (mm)	0.86 ± 0.58	2.62 ± 0.38	1.96 ± 0.69	1.88 ± 0.64
% Stenosis	73 ± 15	15 ± 11	35 ± 20	36 ± 19

Table 3. Stent restenosis as a function of prior PTCA procedures

	Restenosis	
No prior PTCA	12/65 (18%)	$P = 0.05$
1 prior PTCA	20/58 (34%) ⎤	
2 prior PTCA	13/42 (31%) ⎬	$P = NS$
3 prior PTCA	6/16 (38%) ⎦	

as death, myocardial infarction, or urgent bypass surgery occurred in 10 (4.0%) patients.

Results of 4–6 month angiographic core lab analysis vary according to definition. Angiographic restenosis defined as ≥50% narrowing within the stent occurred in 20% of the patients who received single stents and in 50% of those who received multiple stents. Clinical restenosis defined as narrowing in the stent sufficient to cause symptoms or a positive exercise stress test requiring either PTCA or bypass surgery occurred in approximately half of those patients with single stents and angiographic restenosis.

Annual angiography in 31 patients revealed no change in minimal stent lumen diameter when compared with 6-month angiography, 1.96 ± 0.69 mm vs. 1.88 ± 0.64 mm ($P = NS$) (Table 2; personal communication, Michael Savage, M.D.). The influence of prior restenosis on stent restenosis is seen in Table 3 (personal communication, Paul Teirstein, M.D.). Overall, patients who received a single stent at the time of their first angioplasty had a restenosis rate of 18% vs. 34% ($P = 0.05$) when compared with those patients who had one or more prior PTCA procedures. If the group is analyzed by single vs. multiple stents (Table 4), restenosis occurred in 7% vs. 45% ($P < 0.01$). Clinical restenosis occurred in only one patient in the series of patients who received single stents.

A subgroup of 98 patients in the series whose PTCA procedure resulted in a suboptimal angiographic result (defined as the presence of a dissection, filling defect of residual 50% narrowing) has been analyzed with regard to complications (Table 5) and restenosis (Table 6). Subacute closure occurred in 5 patients thus accounting for the majority of thrombotic events within the entire series. Death, myocardial infarction and urgent CABG occurred in 3 (3.2%) of the patients.

Table 4. Influence of prior PTCA on stent restenosis

	Prior restenosis	No prior restenosis
Single stent	25/91 (27%)	3/45 (7%) $P < 0.01$
Multiple stents	14/32 (44%)	9/20 (45%) NS

Table 5. Complications of stenting following "suboptimal PTCA" ($n = 98$ patients)

Acute closure (24 h)	0
Subacute closure (>24 h)	5 (5.1%)
Death	0
Myocardial infarct	3 (3.2%)
Urgent CABG	2 (2.2%)

Table 6. Restenosis following "suboptimal PTCA" ($n = 56$ patients)

	Single	Multiple
Angiographic	7/46 (15%)	7/10 (70%)
Clinical	2/46 (4.3%)	4/10 (40%)

The angiographic restenosis rate in this group of patients was 7/46 (15%) for patients with single stents and 7/10 (70%) for patients who received multiple stents. Clinical restenosis though occurred in 2/46 (4.3%) and 4/10 (40%) in these groups, respectively.

Examples of angiographic outcomes following coronary stenting are seen in Figs. 2–4.

Discussion

Both restenosis and abrupt closure continue to be the two most limiting factors in PTCA today [6–11]. Abrupt closure is a result, generally, of thrombosis, spasm, or dissection following angioplasty. Thus, two of the three causes of abrupt closure are mechanical suggesting that a mechanical prosthesis may solve this problem. Tacking up flaps and improving the flow field may impact thrombosis favorably as well; however, these salutary effects of stenting are offset by the inherent thrombogenicity of most metals. Surface treatment such as polishing, antiplatelet medication, and anti-coagulants appear to solve the immediate thrombosis problem but does not

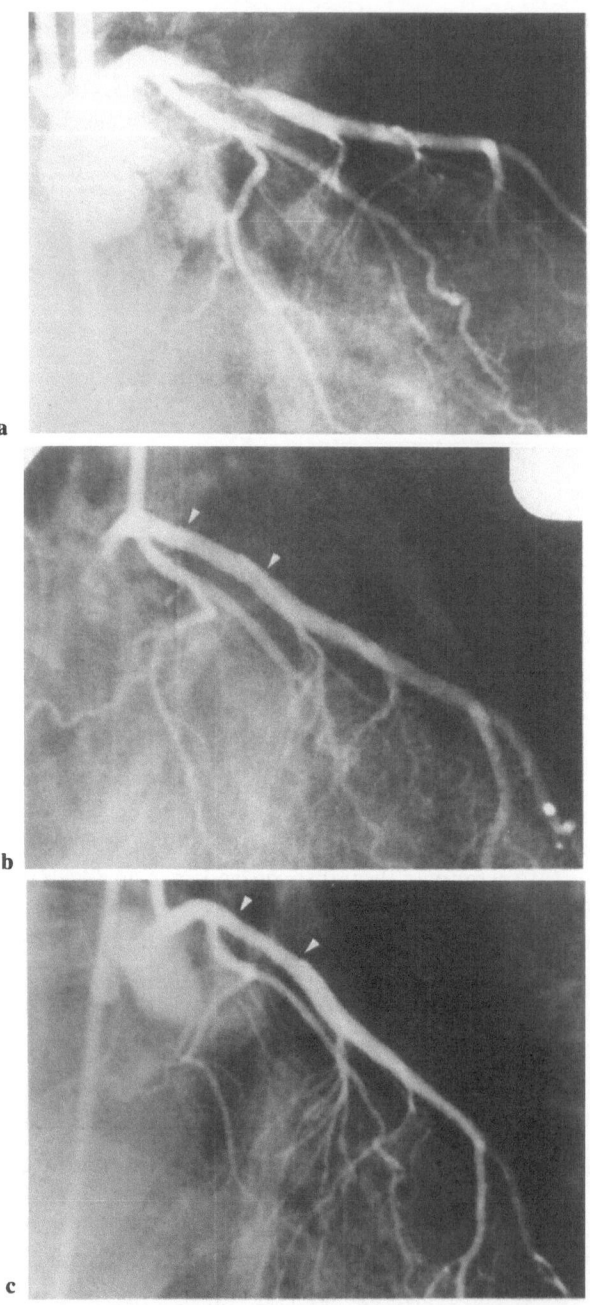

Fig. 2a–c. Angiogram of a 73-year-old woman status post 3 prior PTCA procedures to the LAD (**a**) before stenting, (**b**) immediately after stenting, and (**c**) 6 months post stenting without anticoagulation. *Arrows* indicate stent

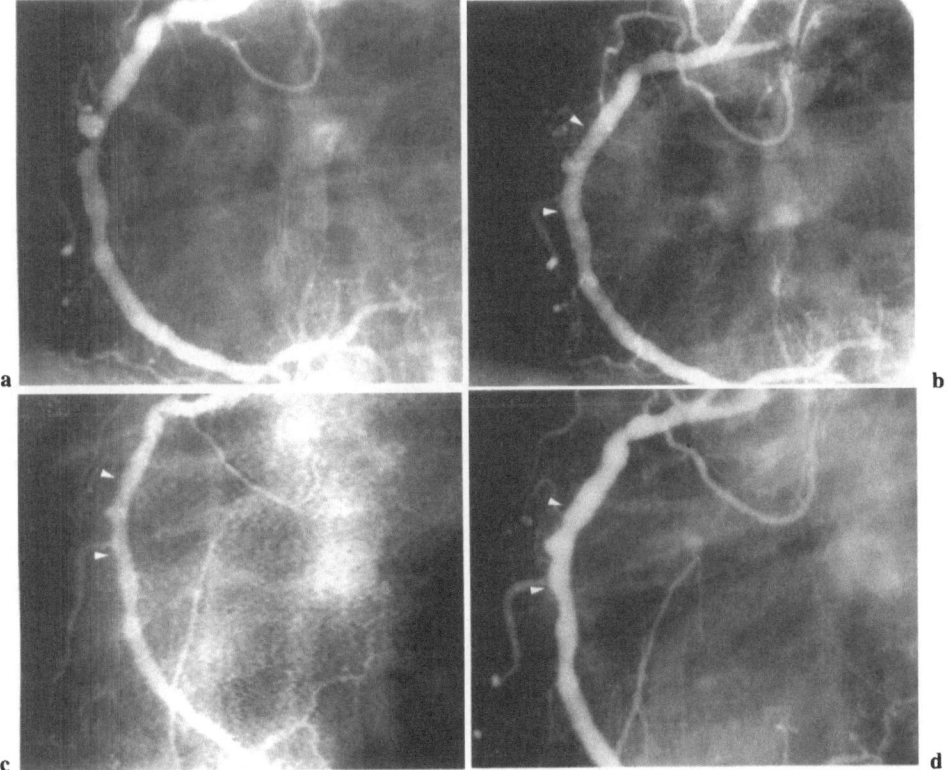

Fig. 3a–d. Angiogram of a 37-year-old man status post 2 prior PTCA procedures to the RCA (**a**) before stenting, (**b**) immediately after stenting, (**c**) 6 months and (**d**) 1 year post stenting with anticoagulation. *Arrows* indicate stent

eliminate delayed thrombosis. This complication introduces a new risk compared with angioplasty since it may occur after hospital discharge. Surface coatings with drugs such as heparin, hirudin, or monoclonal antibodies to specific platelet factors may eliminate this serious complication in the future.

Whether stents reduce restenosis post PTCA can only be answered by carefully planned, randomized controlled studies which are forthcoming. Barring that, one can conclude from our work that at least in a carefully selected patient population that would otherwise be at high risk for restenosis (since 70% of our patients have already failed at least one angioplasty procedure) a restenosis rate of 20% seems quite acceptable. More relevant though is the reduced clinical restenosis rate in these patients. This seemingly low rate of clinical failure is best understood if one analyzes intimal hyperplasia within the stent. Serruys et al. generated a definition of restenosis based upon 0.72 mm of intimal growth within the stent (Wallstent, Lausanne, Switzerland) [12]. If one uses this definition, then 50% of our patients with

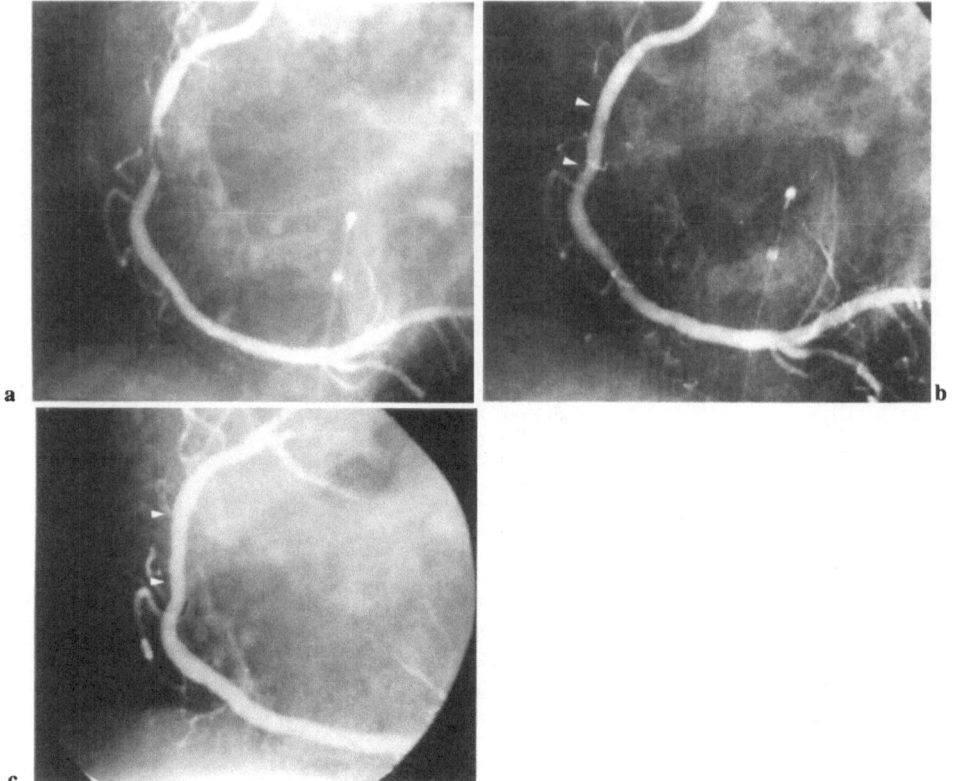

Fig. 4a–c. Angiogram of a 63-year-old woman status post 4 prior PTCA procedures to the RCA (**a**) before stenting, (**b**) immediately after stenting, and (**c**) 1 year post stenting with anticoagulation. *Arrows* indicate stent

single stents developed restenosis (Table 2). However, if one uses greater than 50% lumen stenosis as a definition, then only 20% of the same patients develop restenosis. This observation would suggest that stents do not inhibit smooth muscle cell growth, rather they merely provide an optimal initial lumen diameter so that the usual intimal hyperplasia does not compromise the vessel lumen greater than 50%. More intriguing though is the observation that prior restenosis appears to increase the likelihood of stent restenosis. Experimental models have documented increased smooth muscle cell turn over when endothelial cell cultures are exposed to cyclical trauma [13]. One can speculate that multiple PTCA procedures predispose the target lesion to increased smooth muscle cell growth despite an optimal initial lumen diameter provided by the stent and that perhaps the stent should be placed during the initial angioplasty procedure.

Ellis et al. have provided further evidence that an optimal initial stent lumen diameter is critical to prevent restenosis [14]. In the analysis of single stents, angiographic restenosis occurred in only 14% of patients who left the laboratory with a stent lumen stenosis less than 10% vs. 25% of those patients with a final stent lumen stenosis greater than 10%.

The healing process of the stent has been well documented in multiple animal models and would appear to be complete by 4–6 months [15]. After initial thrombosis fibrin and platelet deposition, fibroblast proliferation seems to peak at approximately 8 weeks. There is gradual thinning of the neointima as the previously cellular infiltrate is replaced with acellular ground substance by 6–8 months. Annual angiography in 31 patients in our series would appear to confirm that the biologic response to these implants is similar in that there is no progression of intimal hyperplasia after 6 months.

The Future

The limitation of this current device gives insight to the future direction of coronary stenting. Subacute thrombosis remains as a serious threat to the ubiquitous application of stents in small vessels and as such much research is being conducted in developing coatings such as heparin, hirudin, or monoclonal antibodies to specific platelet factors to eliminate this complication hopefully. Furthermore, pharmacologic therapy to inhibit smooth muscle cell growth may also be coated onto the stent so that high doses of medications can be concentrated directly at the target site, possibly decreasing the restenosis rate even further.

Radiolucency of the stent remains a problem which may prevent accurate delivery and placement of the stent. Several new metals are being experimented with that will enhance the ability of the operator to see the device during placement. The results of a balloon expandable stent made of tantalum have been previously reported [16].

Conclusions

Despite the absence of randomized controlled studies, this initial report of coronary stenting provides some insight into exciting new technology that may have a great impact on PTCA in the future. In the absence of controlled studies it is reasonable to conclude that: (1) stents can be safely delivered in a high percentage of cases; (2) acute closure due to stent thrombosis within the first 24 h does not occur; (3) subacute thrombosis may occur within the first 2 weeks despite anticoagulation in a small percentage of patients; (4) stenting following suboptimal angioplasty results may be responsible for the larger percentage of subacute thrombosis events suggesting that this subgroup of patients may require adjunctive therapy with thrombolysis at the time of stenting or perhaps during the postoperative period; (5) angiographic restenosis rates appear to be reduced in patients who receive single stents, but especially so in those who receive stents at the time of the first angioplasty; (6) multiple stents are not advised due to the high incidence of restenosis until custom stents of variable lengths become available.

It is hoped that with continuing research future stent design will allow us to conclude that vascular stenting is both a safe and effective approach to the treatment of abrupt closure and restenosis in all patients undergoing PTCA.

References

1. Sigwart U, Urban P, Golf S et al. (1988) Emergency stenting for acute occlusion after coronary balloon angioplasty. Circulation 78:1121–1127
2. Schatz RA (1989) A view of vascular stents. Circulation 79:445–457
3. Palmaz JC, Garcia OJ, Schatz RA et al. (1990) Placement of balloon-expandable intraluminal stents in iliac arteries: first 171 procedures. Radiology 174:969–975
4. Schatz RA, Palmaz JC (1988) Balloon expandable intravascular stents (BEIS) in Human Coronary arteries: report of initial experience. Circulation 78 [Suppl II]:II-415
5. Schatz RA, Leon MB, Baim DS et al. (1989) Balloon expandable intracoronary stents: initial results of a multicenter study. Circulation 80 [Suppl II]:II-174
6. Detre K, Holubkov R, Kelsey S et al. (1988) Co-investigators of the National Heart, Lung, and Blood Institute's percutaneous transluminal coronary angioplasty in 1985–1986 and 1977–1981. N Engl J Med 318:265–270
7. Ellis SG, Roubin GS, King SB III et al. (1988) In-hospital cardiac mortality after acute closure after coronary angioplasty: analysis of risk factors from 8207 procedures. J Am Coll Cardiol 11:211
8. Cowley MJ, Dorros A, Kelsey SF et al. (1984) Acute coronary complications associated with percutaneous transluminal angioplasty. Am J Cardiol 53:12C–16C
9. Ellis SG, Roubin GS, King SB et al. (1988) Angiographic and clinical predictors of acute closure after native vessel coronary angioplasty. Circulation 77:372–379
10. Holmes DR Jr, Vliestra RE, Smith HC et al. (1984) Restenosis after percutaneous transluminal coronary angioplasty (PTCA): a report from the PTCA registry of the National Heart, Lung and Blood Institute. Am J Cardiol 53 [Suppl]:77C–81C
11. Serruys PW, Luitjten HE, Beatt KJ et al. (1988) Incidence of restenosis after successful coronary angioplasty: a time related phenomenon. Circulation 77:361–371
12. Serruys PW, Beatt KJ, van der Giessen WJ (1989) Stenting of coronary arteries. Are we the sorcerer's apprentice? (Editorial.) Eur Heart J 10:774–782
13. Leung DY, Glagov S, Mathews MB (1976) Cyclic stretching stimulates synthesis of matrix components by arterial smooth muscle cells in vitro. Science 191:475
14. Ellis SG, Savage M, Baim D et al. (1990) Intracoronary stenting to prevent restenosis: preliminary results of a multicenter study using the Palmaz-Schatz stent suggest benefit in selected high risk patients. J Am Coll Cardiol 15:118–A

15. Schatz RA, Palmaz JC, Tio FO et al. (1987) Balloon expandable intracoronary stents in the adult dog. Circulation 76:450–457
16. Schatz RA, Palmaz JC, Tio F et al. (1988) Report of a new radiopaque balloon expandable stent (RBEIS) in canine coronary arteries. Circulation 78 [Suppl II]:II-48

Coronary Stenting with the Palmaz-Schatz Stent: The Clinic Pasteur Interventional Cardiology Unit Experience

J. Fajadet, J. Marco, B. Cassagneau, G. Robert, and M. Vandormael[1]

Despite the rapid growth of coronary angioplasty (PTCA) over the past decade and the accompanying improvements in instrumentation and techniques which have improved success and reduced complications, the clinical application of balloon dilatation continues to be tempered by two major shortcomings: abrupt closure, complicating about 5% of procedures, and restenosis, occurring in 25%–50% of patients depending upon the location, the type of occlusion, vessel involved, and the number of lesions dilated [1–5].

Within the past 2–3 years, a variety of diverse new technologies have been developed in an attempt to overcome the limitations of balloon angioplasty. Intracoronary stenting using endovascular metallic stents to support the dilated segment mechanically is one of these new approaches. Although the concept of intravascular stenting was initially introduced by Dotter in the 1960s [6–8], only recently devices have been made available for human coronary evaluation. Three designs of intravascular stents have already undergone relatively large clinical testing: the self-expanding design of Medinvent/Wallstent and the balloon-expandable designs of Palmaz–Schatz and Gianturco Roubin.

It is the purpose of this chapter to summarize and discuss our clinical experience over the past 2 years with intracoronary stenting using the balloon-expandable Palmaz–Schatz stent in an attempt to reduce acute complications and restenosis following coronary angioplasty.

The Device

The Palmaz–Schatz balloon expandable stent (Johnson and Johnson, New Brunswick, NJ) is a relatively rigid slotted tube made of stainless steel. It is 15 mm in length with two 7-mm mesh segments articulated by a 1 mm bridge to increase graft flexibility and permit deployment in tortuous arteries. The

[1] Unité de Cardiologie Interventionnelle, Clinique Pasteur, 45 avenue de Lombez, 31076 Toulouse Cedex, France

Coronary Stents
Edited by U. Sigwart and G.I. Frank
© Springer-Verlag Berlin Heidelberg 1992

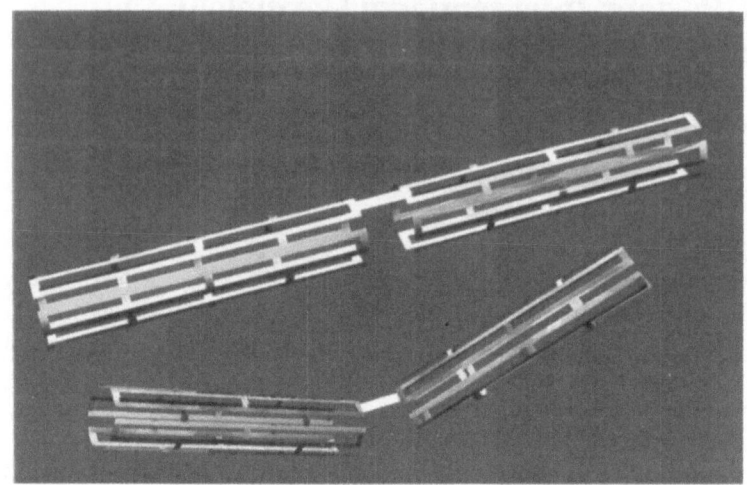

a

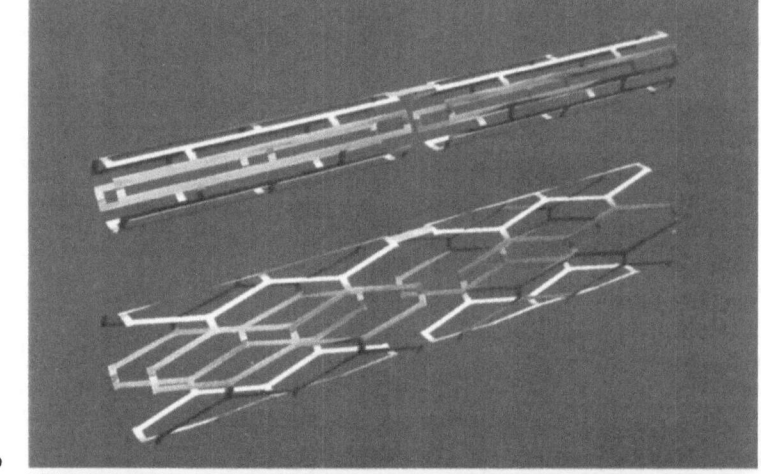

b

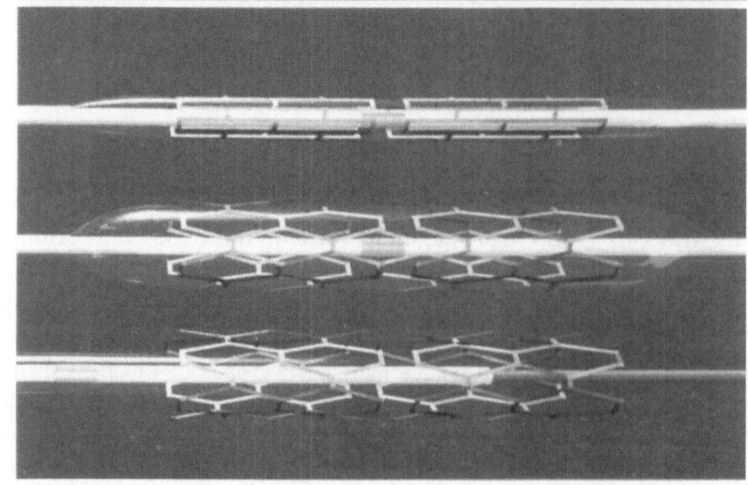

c

collapsed stent diameter is 1.5 mm and can be expanded up to 5 mm. The stent can be mounted on most commercially available angioplasty balloon catheter. Placement in the target site is accomplished by balloon inflation. The principle of the balloon-expandable stent relies on plastic deformation of metal. Once the metal is stretched beyond its elastic limit by balloon inflation, it cannot collapse and remains embedded in the vessel wall (Fig. 1).

Stent Delivery Procedure

The technique of stenting with the Palmaz-Schatz balloon-expandable stent is illustrated in Fig. 2.

The first step in the procedure is to predilate the stenosis with a standard balloon catheter to allow passage of the relatively rigid stent-balloon assembly. This is usually accomplished with a balloon diameter smaller than the diameter of the artery to avoid dissection.

The stent is coaxially mounted on the balloon by crimping it with a specially designed tool. The stent-balloon assembly is introduced into a large lumen guiding catheter and advanced into position over an exchange guide wire across the target area. After assuring the precise position according to vessel landmarks and the balloon catheter marker, the balloon is expanded to its maximal diameter with 10–12 atm of pressure for 20 s. If necessary, the original balloon can be withdrawn and replaced by a larger balloon to expand the graft further. Immediately post placement the stent diameter must be slightly larger than the target vessel in order to accommodate the stent wall thickness and the anticipated intimal growth (stent : artery ratio 1.1–1.2 : 1.0). The balloon and guide wire are removed, leaving the expanded stent firmly embedded in the vessel wall.

Medical Regimen

The drug regimen used for coronary stenting procedures at our institution is based on experimental evidence [9] and early clinical experience [10] demonstrating the role of anticoagulation in preventing stent-associated thrombosis. The day before the procedure aspirin 250 mg p.o. and diltiazem

---

Fig. 1a–c. The Palmaz–Schatz balloon-expandable stent. **a** The articulated design shown unexpanded; **b** stent before and after balloon expansion; **c** stent-balloon apparatus before and after balloon inflation

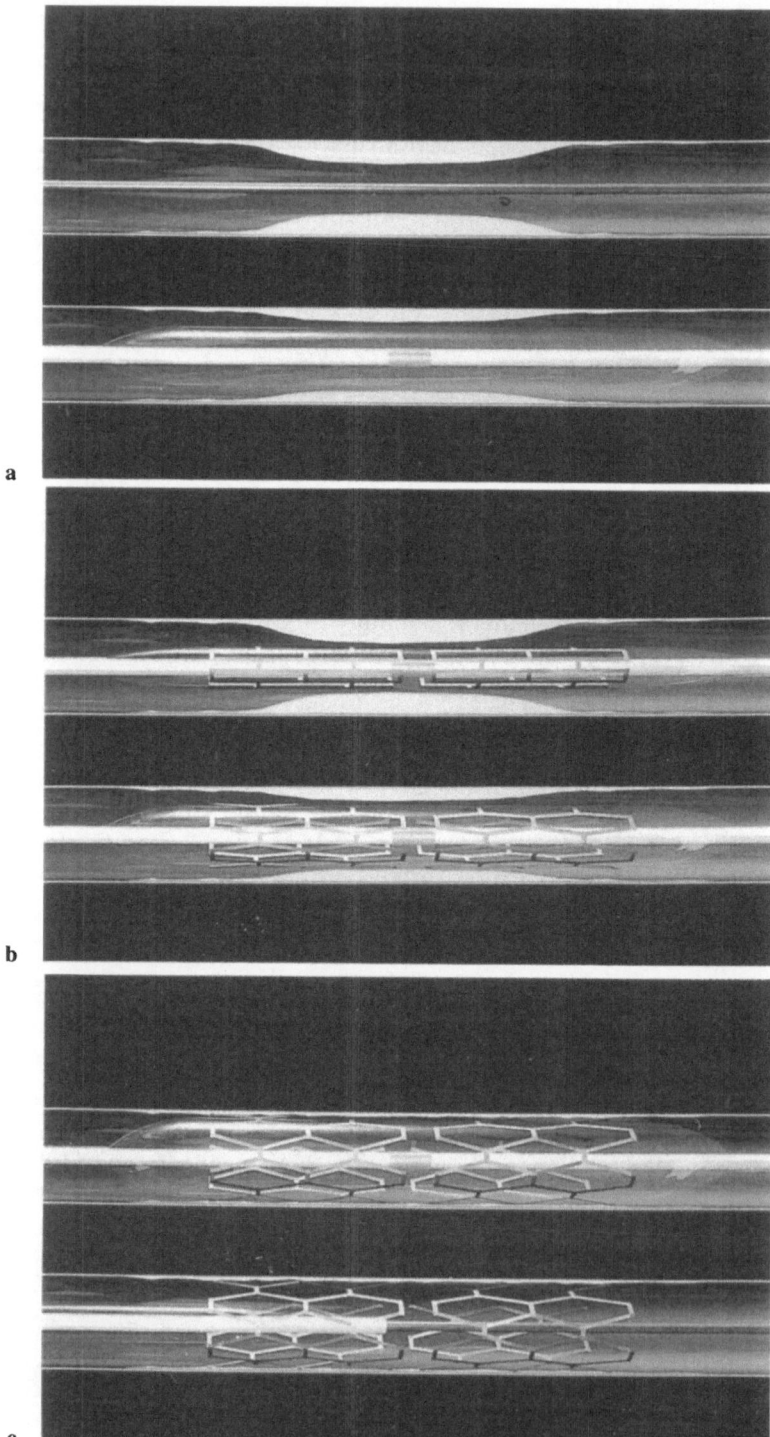

240–360 mg p.o. are administered to the patient. In the laboratory, the patient is sedated with neuroleptanalgesia and aspirin 500 mg bolus i.v., heparin 15 000 units bolus i.v., low molecular weight dextran 500 cc continuous infusion over 6 h, nitroglycerin 0.4 mg intracoronary, and molsidomin 1 mg intracoronary are given prior to stent implantation. Hexabrix is used as the contrast medium. Six hours after the procedure, a continuous heparin infusion is started for 6 days and titrated to maintain an activated partial thromboplastin time (a PTT) between 90 and 120 s. The PTT is checked every 3 h during the first 24 h, every 6 h from days 2 to 4 and twice a day from days 4 to 6. Coumarin derivative is given on day 1 and prescribed for 2 months with prothrombin time maintained at ⩾2.3 the international normalized ratio. Subcutaneous heparin 12 500 units twice a day is administered from days 6 to 12. Aspirin and diltiazem are continued at a daily oral dose of 250 mg and 240–360 mg, respectively.

Table 1. Baseline characteristics of the 290 study patients

Gender (%)	
Male	84
Female	16
Risk factors (%)	
Hypertension	25
Diabetes mellitus	7
Hypercholesterolemia	30
Smoking	49
Family history of CAD	11
Cardiac history (%)	
Silent ischemia	4
Stable angina	46
Unstable angina	48
Acute myocardial infarction	2
Prior PTCA	28
Prior coronary surgery	11
Prior myocardial infarction	25
Mean age (years, range)	59 (30–77)
Mean LVEF (%, range)	58 (20–75)
Extend of CAD (%)	
1 vessel disease	54
2 vessel disease	28
3 vessel disease	18

CAD, coronary artery disease; LVEF, left ventricular ejection fraction.

←

Fig. 2a–c. Procedure of implantation of the Palmaz–Schatz stent. **a** Predilatation of the stenosis with a standard balloon catheter; **b** the stent-balloon apparatus is centered in the stenosis, and the stent is released by balloon inflation; **c** the stent is further expanded with a larger balloon size and then left firmly embedded in the vessel wall

Table 2. Indications for coronary stenting (n = 290 patients)

Indication	No. of patients
Balloon angioplasty restenosis	81 (28%)
First restenosis	75
Second restenosis	6
PTCA in "high restenosis risk" lesion	128 (44%)
Chronic total occlusion	16
Proximal left anterior descending artery stenosis	56
Body of saphenous vein graft	20
Variant angina and/or subtotal lesion	36
Abrupt closure or suboptimal PTCA result	81 (28%)
Acute closure	23
Suboptimal PTCA result	58

The femoral arterial sheath is removed the morning following the procedure. Intravenous heparin is usually stopped for 1 h before sheath removal and resumed immediately after hemostasis has been obtained.

Study Patients

Between March 1989 and October 1990, we attempted intracoronary placement of a Palmaz–Schatz stent in 290 patients drawn from 2165 patients who underwent coronary angioplasty during the same period at our institution. The study population consisted of 244 men and 46 women whose mean age was 59 years (range 30–77 years). Baseline clinical and angiographic characteristics are summarized in Table 1. Some 28% of the patients had a history of prior balloon angioplasty, 48% presented with unstable angina, 46% had either two or three vessel coronary disease. The mean left ventricular ejection fraction was 58% (range 20%–75%). Patients were selected (Table 2) on the basis of three major indications for coronary stenting:

1. *Restenosis after balloon angioplasty*: for 81 patients (28%) of whom 6 had developed a second restenosis
2. *High restenosis risk lesion* (Figs. 3, 4): for 128 patients (44%); the type of occlusion or vessel, the location, and the lesion characteristics were felt to be at high risk for restenosis

Fig. 3a–c. Coronary stenting with Palmaz–Schatz stent of a chronic total occlusion after successful balloon recanalization. **a** Chronic total occlusion of a right coronary artery; **b** successful balloon recanalization and implantation of a Palmaz–Schatz stent; **c** 5-month follow-up angiogram

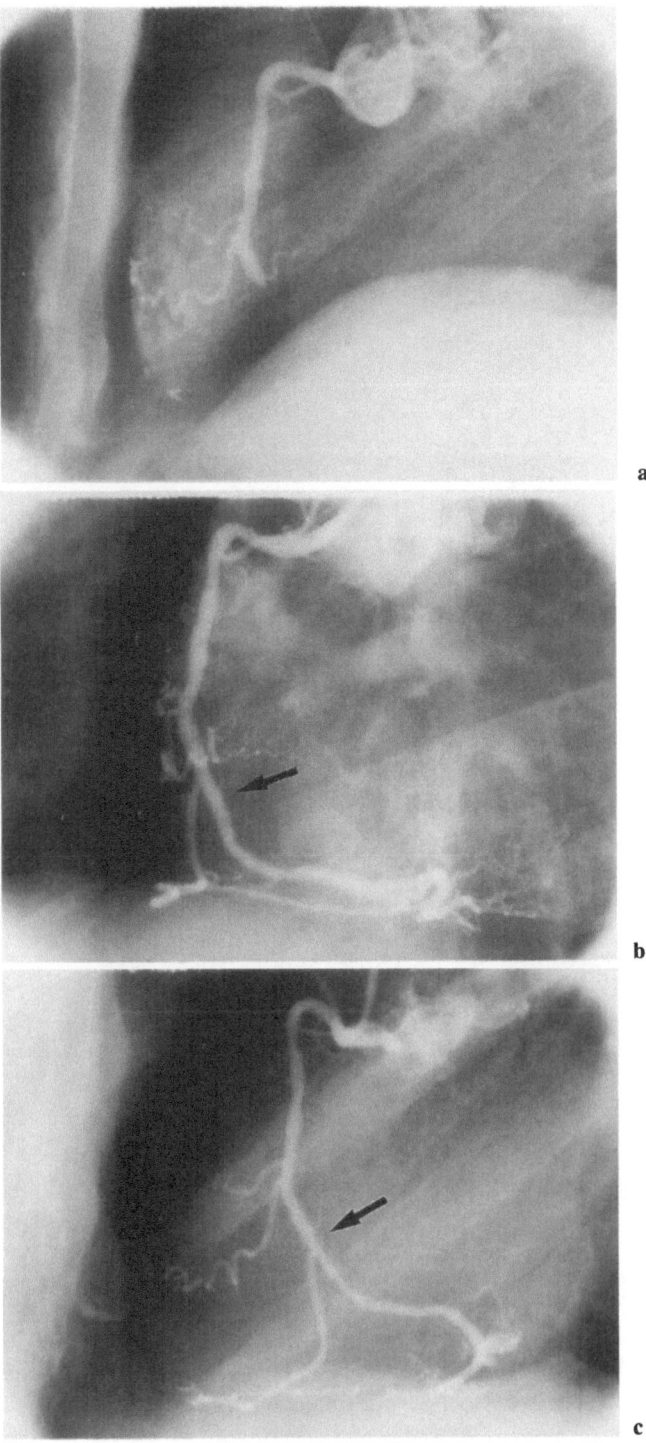

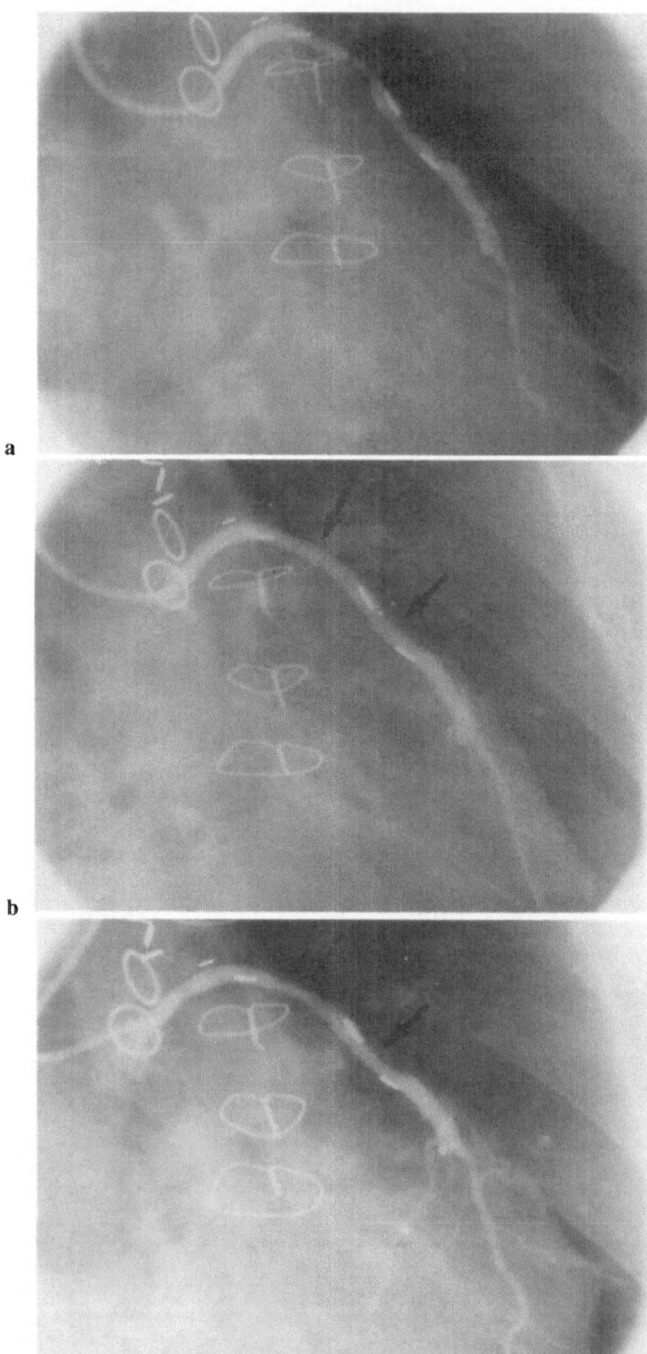

a

b

c

3. *Treatment of abrupt closure or suboptimal PTCA result* (Fig. 5): for 81 patients (28%) of whom 23 had abrupt closure and 58 had a suboptimal PTCA result (defined as the presence of a linear or complex dissection or the persistence of ⩾50% luminal diameter narrowing)

Immediate Results

Stent placement was technically successful in 284 (98%) of the 290 patients. Failure to deliver the stent to the target lesion occurred in 6 patients due to the inability to reach or pass the stent across the lesion. Failed delivery resulted from snagging of the stent-balloon assembly on proximal diffuse calcific disease in 2 patients, from severe proximal tortuosity with a shepherd cross morphology in 2 patients and from poor guiding catheter support in saphenous vein graft in 2 patients. All 6 patients were successfully dilated by conventional balloon angioplasty.

Stent detachment and embolization into the peripheral circulation occurred during attempted withdrawal in 4 patients without sequelae.

Overall 340 stents were implanted in 294 vessels of 284 patients. The vessel involved was the left anterior descending artery in 136 patients, the right coronary artery in 87 patients, the left circumflex artery in 51 patients, and a saphenous vein graft in 20 patients. Some 240 patients (85%) received a single stent, 37 received 2, 3 received 3, 3 received 4, and 1 received 5 stents. Among the 44 patients who had multiple stents, 35 had the stents placed contiguously in the same vessel, and 9 patients had the multiple stents placed in different vessels.

The final stent diameter measured by balloon size at maximal balloon inflation was ⩽3.0 mm in 71 implants and ⩾3.1 mm in 269 implants. Stent deployment resulted in widely patent vessels with a residual diameter stenosis within the stented segment of less than 10% in all patients.

Patients stented for abrupt closure had few complications during the hospital stay. PTCA flow limiting dissections were abolished in all 23 patients who underwent coronary stenting as a bail-out procedure with immediate relief from chest pain and correction of ischemic EKG changes. Despite successful stenting, 2 of these patients suffered a moderate rise in cardiac enzymes, and 3 developed a Q wave infarction. There was no death

←

Fig. 4a–c. Double Palmaz–Schatz stent placement in a saphenous vein graft. **a** Angiogram before balloon angioplasty shows two stenoses of a 4-year-old vein graft to the left anterior descending artery; **b** successful angiographic result after implantation of two stents (*arrows*); **c** 6-month follow-up angiogram reveals absence of restenosis in the stented segments (*arrows*)

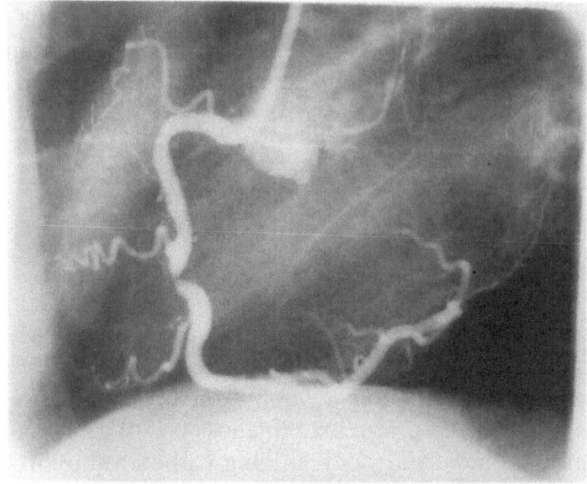

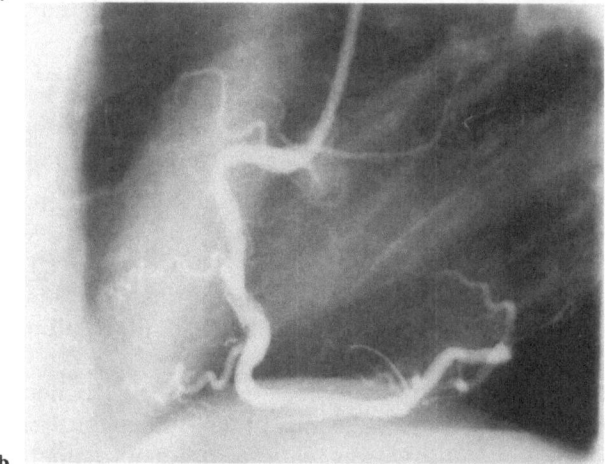

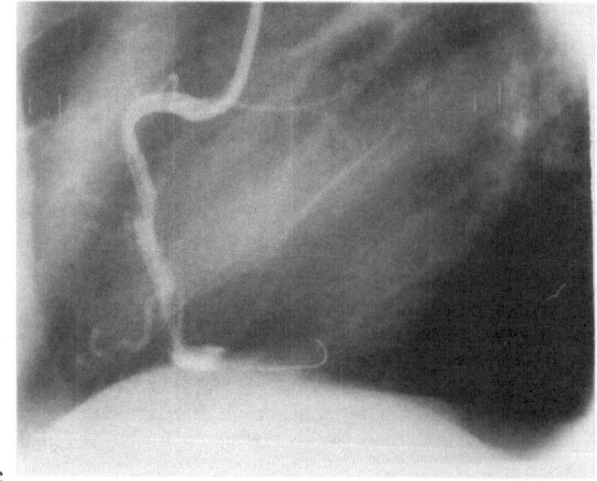

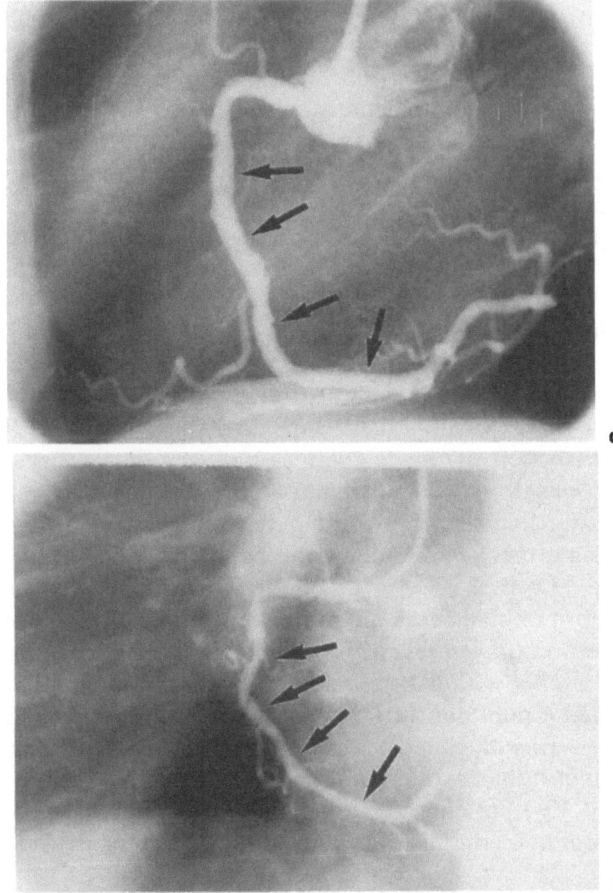

Fig. 5a–e. Multiple Palmaz–Schatz stent implantation for the treatment of an occlusive right coronary artery dissection (emergency bail-out procedure). **a** Angiogram shows a severe, eccentric stenosis of the mid-right coronary artery before PTCA; **b** large dissection following the first balloon inflation; **c** dissection has extended distally and progressed to abrupt closure; **d** immediate angiographic result after the implantation of four stents in tandem; **e** repeat angiography 6 months later shows a good patency of the right coronary artery with no restenosis

and no patient requiring emergency bypass surgery in this subgroup of patients.

Stenting related complications occurred *during the procedure or within the first 24 h* in 2 patients (1%). Both patients required emergency bypass surgery because of severe ischemia due to an ostial guiding catheter dissection in one patient and to acute thrombosis of an underexpanded stent at a bend point lesion in the other patient. One patient underwent the same day elective coronary surgery because of an incomplete correction of a large dissection with a single stent and did not have ischemic complications.

From day 2 to hospital discharge, 6 patients (2%) developed ischemic symptoms due to acute stent thrombosis. In 5 there was a complete occlusion of the stented segment which was acutely recanalized by repeat dilatation and/or intracoronary thrombolysis without a myocardial infarction in 3 patients and with a Q wave myocardial infarction in 1 patient. This latter patient had a bail-out stenting procedure. One patient could not be recanalized and died 6 days later from a large anterior infarction. The sixth patient had only a subtotal occlusion (filling defects) of the stented area, and he was successfully redilated with no evidence of myocardial necrosis.

From hospital discharge to 1 month after implantation, 3 additional patients developed an acute thrombotic occlusion of the stented vessel. Two of these patients died. One had received three stents for a long occlusive dissection of the left anterior descending artery, and the other one had a poor left ventricular function and a single stent placed to his only remaining patent vessel. The third patient developed a myocardial infarction despite acute mechanical reopening of the occluded vessel.

Overall 272 (96%) of the 284 patients who had a technically successful stent implantation did not have complications. Major complications (Q wave infarction, emergency bypass surgery, and death) occurred in 3.5% of the patients within the first month after stent implantation: 7 patients (2.5%) had a nonfatal thrombotic event, and 3 patients (1%) died.

Bleeding and vascular complications (large groin hematoma and false aneurysm of the femoral artery) requiring surgical repair occurred in 13 (4.5%) patients. These events were related to the aggressive anticoagulant regimen administered during the poststent period.

Follow-up

Clinical follow-up (clinic visit or telephone contact) of the 272 patients with successful stent placement and no complications has ranged from 1 to 18 months (mean 8.3 months) post placement. During the follow-up period cardiac events occurred in 30 patients: 2 patients died suddenly, 1 patient had a nonfatal myocardial infarction, 21 patients underwent repeat PTCA, 1 patient had a directional atherectomy, and 5 patients had coronary bypass surgery. Some 242 (89%) patients remained free of cardiac events; of these patients 6 were symptomatic with Canadian Heart Association angina class ≥II, and 236 were asymptomatic or had angina class I.

Angiographic follow-up (mean 4.2 months, range 1–13 months) was achieved in 173 (84%) of the 207 eligible patients for the routine 4–6 month restudy. Of the asymptomatic patients 32 refused repeat catheterization, and 2 patients were lost to follow-up.

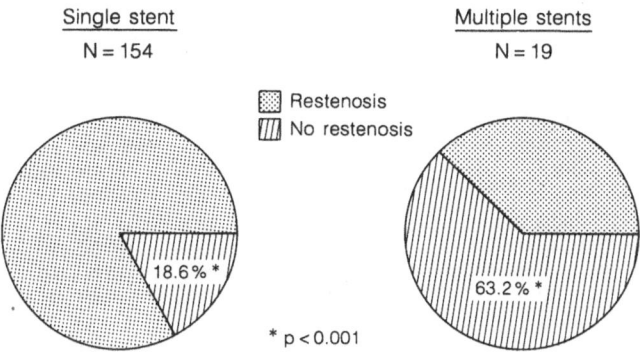

Fig. 6. Angiographic restenosis rate following Palmaz–Schatz stent implantation in 173 patients (mean follow-up 4.2 months)

Restenosis defined as ≥50% luminal diameter narrowing within the stented segment (visual interpretation) was observed in 41 patients (24%).

Following single-stent implantation, restenosis occurred in 29 of 154 patients (19%). After multiple contiguous stent placement the restenosis rate was 63% (12/19 patients) which was statistically greater than after single-stent implantation (19% versus 63%, $P < 0.001$) (Fig. 6).

Among the 29 patients with single-stent placement who developed restenosis, 7 patients were asymptomatic with a normal stress thallium scintigraphy and a <70% restenosis. These patients were managed medically. The 22 symptomatic patients had either a ≥70% restenosis (20 patients) or a total occlusion (2 patients). Of the 20 patients with restenosis, 4 underwent coronary bypass surgery, 15 had repeat angioplasty, and 1 underwent directional atherectomy. Of the 2 patients who developed a total occlusion, 1 had a successful mechanical recanalization, and 1 was medically treated.

The restenosis rate was slightly higher for stents implanted in the left anterior descending artery (23%) and saphenous vein graft (20%) as compared with left circumflex artery (14%) or right coronary artery (12.5%) implantations, but these differences were not statistically significant.

A univariate analysis of 11 clinical and 7 angiographic variables found that a history of smoking, unstable angina, male gender and one angiographic variable, the final diameter of the prosthesis (stent size), were significant predictors of restenosis after single stent coronary placement (Table 3).

The restenosis rate was 28% for a stent size of ≤3.0 mm compared with 15% for a stent size of ≥3.1 mm ($P < 0.02$) (Table 4). Patients stented for restenosis had a 24% restenosis rate, not significantly different from the rate of restenosis (18%) in patients with no prior angioplasty.

Table 3. Predictors of restenosis by univariate analysis following successful single-stent placement in 154 patients (restenosis rate)

Clinical variable	Present	Absent	P value
Smoking	28%	13%	<0.02
Diabetes	29%	18%	NS
Age >60 years	23%	16%	NS
Hypertension	28%	19%	NS
Hypercholesterolemia	17%	20%	NS
Male gender	22%	4%	<0.02
Indication for restenosis	24%	17%	NS
Unstable angina	26%	13%	<0.02

Table 4. Predictors of restenosis by univariate analysis following successful single-stent placement in 160 vessels

Angiographic variables		Restenosis rate	P value
Vessels			
Left anterior descending artery	(17/73)	23.3% ⎫	
Left circumflex artery	(4/29)	13.8% ⎪	
Right coronary artery	(6/48)	12.5% ⎬	NS
Saphenous vein graft	(2/10)	20.0% ⎭	
Stent diameter			
≤3.0 mm	(11/40)	28% ⎫	
≥3.1 mm	(18/120)	15% ⎭	<0.02

Discussion

Intravascular stents are scaffolding devices designed to support the vessel wall mechanically after balloon deflation, thus preventing collapse or elastic recoil of the dilated segment. Experimental and animal studies [11–16] as well as clinical studies in human peripheral circulation [17, 18] have shown that by tacking-up plaque fragments and by optimising stenosis geometry and luminal surface these devices are effective in improving immediate balloon angioplasty results and appear a promising solution to reduce or prevent acute complications and restenosis associated with balloon angioplasty.

Initial clinical experience with coronary stenting [11, 19–22] has highlighted a variety of problems regarding ease of deployment, propensity for thrombosis, and gradual restenosis from neointimal hyperplasia within the stented area. These problems have varied in importance with the specific stent characteristics which influence device flexibility and biocompatibility.

Each stent design currently undergoing clinical testing is a metallic (stainless steel or metal alloy) foreign body with its own particular advantages and problems. No device appears clearly superior.

Our experience with coronary stenting began in March 1989 and has only involved the use of the Palmaz–Schatz articulated design. At the time of this writing approximately, 350 patients have had one or more stents implanted at our institution. The data presented in this chapter concern immediate and follow-up results of the first 290 patients. Our study population consisted of two types of patients: those in whom a stent was implanted electively for the treatment or prevention of restenosis (72%) and those who were stented for the treatment of an occlusive dissection (abrupt closure) or of a suboptimal angioplasty result (28%). The majority of patients received a single stent. Multiple stents were placed in 15% of the patients, but multiple contiguous stent placement was performed only for stenting of extensive dissection.

The procedure of stent implantation itself has not been source of great technical difficulties and with experience the procedure takes less than 20 min once the initial balloon dilatation has been completed. Angiographic evaluation after technically successful stent placement consistently showed improved initial angiographic result compared with that of balloon dilatation alone with a final luminal diameter narrowing of the stented segment less than 10% in all patients.

Ease of Stent Delivery

In this series all stents were delivered crimped onto a low profile balloon catheter (LPS, USCI; ACX, ACS; RX, ACS; Piccolino Schneider). The new sheated delivery system was not used. Failure to deliver the stent to the target lesion occurred in only 2% of patients but did not cause complications. Severe tortuosity of the vessel to be implanted, diffuse calcific disease in segments proximal to the lesion, target stenosis located at a bend point ≥45°, and poor guiding catheter support were the reasons for technical failures. The balloon-stent assembly is much stiffer and has a rather rough surface, making the apparatus less flexible and less trackable than most commercially available catheters.

Although firmly mounted on the balloon, the stent may strip off and embolize. In our series no stent migration occurred into the coronary circulation, and no clinical adverse consequenses resulted from peripheral embolization. Stent detachment occurred during unsuccessful stent delivery upon removal of the stent-balloon apparatus or after forceful maneuvers to advance the stent-balloon assembly through tortuous or diffusely diseased proximal segments. Despite improved flexibility, the articulated design still poses difficulties in placement, and careful patient selection with appropriate anatomy and optimal choice of equipment are of significant importance to

Table 5. Contraindications coronary stenting with Palmaz–Schatz stent

---

Anatomical contraindications
Vessel diameter <3.0 mm
Severe tortuosity in proximal segment
Diffuse disease and calcifications in proximal segment
Lesion at bend point >45°
Severely calcified or poorly expandable lesion
Lesion with filling defect
Large side branch in the segment to be stented
Lesion length >15 mm
Poor distal runoff

Clinical contraindications
Any contraindication or anticipated difficulty with the antiplatelet and anticoagulation
regimen

---

facilitate stent deployment (Table 5). These problems should be partially
eliminated by the use of a new sheated delivery system. Preliminary experience [23] with this new system demonstrated excellent maneuverability
and virtually eliminated undesired proximal deployment or embolization.

Complications

Although the animal studies [13, 15, 16] and the clinical studies in the
peripheral circulation [18] have indicated that the Palmaz–Schatz stent is
relatively nonthrombogenic, its metallic nature makes it inherently thrombogenic until it is completely covered by a thin neointimal layer, which usually
takes a few weeks. Therefore, anticoagulant therapy is mandatory to prevent
thrombotic occlusion for several weeks after implantation.

During the first month after stent implantation, acute thrombotic occlusion of the stented segment occurred in 3.5% of our patients despite a
regimen of heparin, dextran, aspirin, and oral anticoagulant.

The majority (70%) of these thrombotic events occurred during hospital stay and were managed by repeat dilatation and intracoronary thrombolytic therapy (urokinase). Retrospective analysis allowed us to identify
a "predisposing" cause in all but one of the patients who developed a
thrombotic occlusion: undersized stent placed at a bend point, evidence of
intraluminal thrombus prior to stent placement, residual narrowing at a
stent extremity (inflow or outflow obstruction), poor distal runoff, and
aspirin discontinuation.

Overall, an acceptably low complication rate was observed, with a 1%
mortality rate and less than 1% incidence of myocardial infarction and need
for emergency bypass surgery during the first month after implantation.

Table 6. Stent-related major complications within 30 days after technically successful implantation

Indication	Major complications	
	MI, emergency CABG	Death
Elective stenting	4/203 (2.0%)	1/203 (0.5%)
Unsatisfactory result or abrupt closure	3/81 (3.7%)	2/81 (2.5%)

MI, myocardial infarction; CABG, coronary artery bypass graft surgery.

Although this is not negligible, it compares favorably with conventional balloon angioplasty results [1].

In our experience complications occurred more frequently in the group of patients who were stented acutely for abrupt closure or suboptimal angioplasty results as compared to the group of patients who were electively stented (Table 6). When treating long occlusive dissection, close attention must be paid to ensure that the dissection is completely covered by the prosthesis because incomplete correction of the dissection predisposes to abrupt closure.

In addition to a strict monitoring of the anticoagulant therapy, proper patient selection and a meticulous angiographic examination at the completion of the procedure, particularly in regards to any potential limitation of flow through the stented segment, are critical to avoid thrombotic complications.

The importance of the learning curve in patient selection and methodology has been underlined by Sigwart et al. [24]. Using the self-expand-

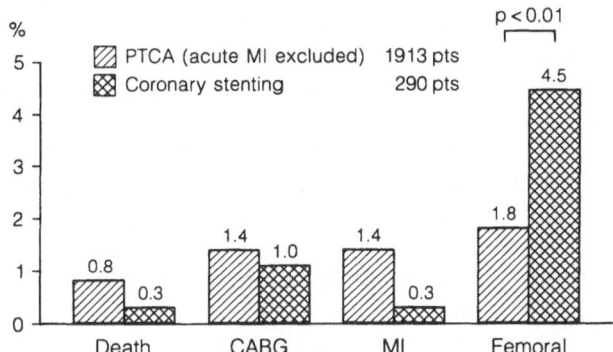

Fig. 7. Comparison of in-hospital complications between balloon angioplasty and coronary stenting, March 1989–October 1990. *CABG*, coronary artery bypass graft surgery; *MI*, Myocardial infarction

able Medinvent stent they observed a decrease from 14% to 6% in the incidence of thrombotic occlusion between their early and more recent experience.

Bleeding and local vascular complications at the arterial puncture site occurred more frequently than after balloon angioplasty as a consequence of the anticoagulant regimen (Fig. 7). Approximately 5% of our patients required blood transfusion or surgical repair. However, these local complications did not compromise stent patency nor cardiac status but resulted in a longer hospital stay. In an attempt to reduce bleeding complications, we now remove the arterial sheath 4–6 h after the procedure before starting the heparin infusion.

Restenosis

In this series of patients with a relatively high restudy rate (84%), the overall 6-month angiographic restenosis rate was 24%, which does not seem at first to be different from that reported after balloon angioplasty alone. However, subgroup analysis showed that patients with multiple contiguous stents had a high recurrence rate (63%), and in contrast the restenosis rate following a single stent procedure was only 19%. This low incidence of restenosis after single-stent implantation is quite favorable considering that approximately two-thirds of the patients were initially selected because they were at high risk for restenosis and considering that all patients not restudied were asymptomatic at 6 months therefore producing a bias towards a higher restenosis rate. In this series only 6% of asymptomatic patients at a time of restudy had evidence of angiographic restenosis.

The prohibitive restenosis rate observed in patients who received multiple contiguous stents may be explained in part by the increased concentration of metal at the overlapping extremities of the stents. Animal studies [25] have shown that this may cause increased focal thrombus deposition and neointimal proliferation. With the current poorly radioopaque design, multiple-stent placement must be avoided and reserved only for correction of long dissection compromising coronary flow (bail-out situation).

We observed a relationship between the final stent diameter and the incidence of restenosis. With a stent size equal or greater than 3.1 mm, the incidence of restenosis dropped significantly (15%).

Similar findings have been reported by Ellis et al. [26] who observed with the same stent design that the incidence of restenosis was highly dependent in multivariate analysis on the number of stents per stenosis placed and the final stent diameter <3.2 mm. Correction of the flow disturbances and shear forces may be greater in larger vessels, further reducing contact of blood elements and mural thrombosis, thereby setting optimal conditions for limited intimal growth. When stenting for prevention of restenosis is contemplated, vessel size greater than 3.0 mm must be a major consideration in patient selection. Restenosis within the stented area has been amenable to repeat angioplasty. Fifteen patients with symptomatic restenosis were successfully redilated. Clinical follow-up of these patients is favorable with 13 patients asymptomatic at last contact. Only 2 patients became symptomatic and required another procedure. Additional data are needed to determine whether repeat angioplasty of stented segment have a good long-term prognosis.

Conclusion

Our experience with the Palmaz–Schatz balloon-expandable coronary stent is encouraging and suggests that in carefully selected patients intravascular stents may represent a valuable adjunct to balloon angioplasty. Stents appear to provide an effective alternative to emergency bypass surgery in many cases for management of abrupt closure. Coronary stenting improves the efficacy of balloon angioplasty and appears to alter favorable the restenosis rate.

However, with the currently available stent designs, several problems need to be solved before widespread clinical use could be recommended. Improvements in the flexibility and visibility is needed to facilitate stent implantation. New types of metal and new delivery systems are being developed to overcome these problems. Despite a complex and aggressive anticoagulant regimen, abrupt thrombotic occlusion still occurs and remains the "Achilles heel" of this technique responsible for most of the major complications. Further work is required to develop means to reduce stent thrombogenicity. This problem is currently being approached by coating the metallic stents with polymers or heparin and by the development of bio-degradable polymeric stents. Clinical implication of long-term placement of prosthetic metallic devices into coronary arteries remains unknown. In conjunction with improved stent characteristics to facilitate implantation and to decrease thrombotic complications, new pharmacological approaches to the control of thrombosis and intimal proliferation should advance the practice of coronary stenting and interventional cardiology.

References

1. Holmes DR, Holubkov R, Vliestra RE, Kelsey SF, Reeder GS, Dorros G, William DO, Cowley MJ, Faxon DP, Kent KM, Bentivoglio LG, Detre K (1988) Co-investigators of the NHLBI PTCA Registry: comparison of complications during percutaneous transluminal coronary angioplasty from 1977 to 1981 and from 1985 to 1986: the National Heart, Lung and Blood Institute percutaneous transluminal coronary angioplasty registry. J Am Coll Cardiol 12:1149–1155
2. Detre KM, Holmes DR, Holubkov R, Cowley MJ, Bourassa MG, Faxon DP, Dorros GR, Bentivoglio LG, Kent KM, Myler RK (1990) Coinvestigators of the National Heart, Lung and Blood Institute's percutaneous transluminal coronary angioplasty registry: incidence and consequences of periprocedural occlusion. The 1985–1986 National Heart, Lung, and Blood Institute percutaneous transluminal coronary angioplasty registry. Circulation 82:739–750
3. Ellis SG, Roubin GS, King SB III, Douglas JS, Weintraub WS, Thomas RG, Cos WR (1988) Angiographic and clinical predictors of acute closure after native vessel coronary angioplasty. Circulation 77:372–379
4. Leimgruber PP, Roubin GS, Hollman J, Cotsonis GA, Meier B, Douglas JS, King SB, Gruentzig AR (1986) Restenosis after successful coronary angioplasty in patients with single-vessel disease. Circulation 73:710–717
5. Holmes DR, Vliestra RE, Smith HC, Vetrovec GW, Kent KM, Cowley MJ, Faxon DP, Gruentzig AR, Kelsey SF, Detre KM, Van Raden MJ, Mock MB (1984) Restenosis after percutaneous transluminal coronary angioplasty (PTCA): a report from the PTCA registry of the National Heart, Lung, and Blood Institute. J Am Coll Cardiol 53:77C–81C
6. Dotter CT, Judkins MP (1964) Transluminal treatment of atherosclerotic obstruction description of a new technique and preliminary report of its application. Circulation 30:654–670
7. Dotter CT, Buschmann RW, McKinney MK, Rosch J (1983) Transluminal expandable nitinol coil stent grafting: preliminary report. Radiology 147:259–260
8. Dotter CT (1969) Transluminally-placed coilspring endarterial tube grafts: long-term patency in canine popliteal artery. Invest Radiol 4:329–332
9. Palmaz JC, Garcia OJ, Copp DT et al. (1987) Balloon expandable intra-arterial stents: effect of anticoagulation on thrombus formation (abstract). Circulation 76: IV-45
10. Schatz RA, Leon MB, Baim DS, Ellis SG, Erbel R, Hirshfeld JW, Goldberg S, Penn IM (1989) Balloon expandable intracoronary stents: initial results of a multicenter study. Circulation 80:II-174
11. Sigwart U, Puel J, Mirkowitch V, Joffre F, Kappenbergen L (1987) Intravascular stents to prevent occlusion and restenosis after transluminal angioplasty. N Engl J Med 316:701
12. Palmaz JC, Sibbitt RR, Reuter SR, Tio FO, Rice WJ (1985) Expandable intraluminal graft: preliminary study. Radiology 156:73
13. Palmaz JC, Windelar SA, Garcia F, Tio FO, Sibbitt RR, Reuter SR (1986) Balloon expandable intraluminal grafting of atherosclerotic rabbit aortas. Radiology 160:723
14. Palmaz JC, Kopp DT, Harashi H, Schatz RA, Hunter G, Tio FO, Garcia O, Alvarado R, Rees C, Thomas SC (1987) Normal and stenotic renal arteries: experimental balloon expandable intraluminal stenting. Radiology 164:705
15. Schatz RA, Palmaz C, Tio FO, Garcia F, Garcia O, Reuter SR (1987) Balloon expandable intracoronary stents in the adult dog. Circulation 76:450
16. Schatz RA, Tio F, Palmaz JC, Garcia O (1987) Balloon expandable intravascular stents in deceased human cadaver coronary arteries (abstract). Circulation 76:IV-26
17. Palmaz JC, Richter G, Noeldge G, Schatz RA, Robison P, Gardiner G, Becker G, McLean G, Denny DF, Lammer J, Paolini R, Rees C, Alvarado R, Heiss HW, Root

H, Rogers W (1988) Intraluminal stents in Atherosclerotic iliac artery stenosis: preliminary report of a multicenter study. Radiology 168:727–731

18. Palmaz JC, Schatz RA, Richter G, Gardiner G, Becker G, Garcia O (1988) Intraluminal stenting of iliac artery stenosis: preliminary report of a multicenter study. Circulation 78:II-415
19. Sigwart U, Golf S, Kaufman U, Kappenberger L (1988) Analysis of complications associated with coronary stenting (abstract). J Am Coll Cardiol 11:66A
20. Baim DS, Schatz RA, Cleman M, Curry C (1989) Predictors of unsuccessful placement of the Schatz-Palmaz coronary stent. Circulation 80:II-174
21. Leon MB, Almagor Y, Erbel R, Teirstein PS, Perez J, Schatz RA (1989) Subacute thrombotic events after coronary stent placement: clinical spectrum and predictive factors. Circulation 80:II-174
22. Serruys PW, Beatt KJ, Bertrand M, Meier B, Puel J, Rickards T, Sigwart U (1989) Restenosis rate after coronary stent implantation. Angiographic assessment of the initial series. Circulation 80:II-173
23. Baim DS, Bailey S, Curry C, Walker C, Schatz RA (1990) Improved success and safety of Palmaz-Schatz coronary stenting with a new delivery system. Circulation 82:III-657
24. Sigwart U, Urban P, Sadeghi H, Kappenberger L (1989) Implantation of 100 intracoronary stents. Learning curve effect on the occurence of acute complications (abstract). J Am Coll Cardiol 13:107A
25. Schatz RA (1989) A view of vascular stents. Circulation 79:445–457
26. Ellis SG, Savage M, Baim D, Hirshfeld J, Cleman M, Teirstein P, Topol EJ (1990) Intracoronary stenting to prevent restenosis: preliminary results of a multicenter study using the Palmaz-Schatz stent suggest benefit in selected high risk patients. J Am Coll Cardiol 15, 2:118A

Gianturco-Roubin Stent: Development and Investigation

G.S. Roubin[1] and C.A. Pinkerton[2]

> If I set out to prove something, I am no real scientist –
> I have to learn to follow where the facts lead me –
> I have to learn to whip my prejudices.
>
> Spallanzani
> 1729–1799

> Medicine requires not only the intellectual cultivation of a
> science, but the patience and practical skills of an art.
>
> Sir William Gull
> The Study of Medicine, 1855

History and Development

The stent was designed specifically to act as an intra-arterial "scaffold" in cases of acute closure following coronary angioplasty. The balloon-expandable coil concept was initially conceived by Cesare Gianturco at M.D. Anderson Hospital in 1983. Modifications to Gianturco's design were undertaken by Roubin (1985) when intracoronary animal studies began. After investigating a range of metallic fibers, stainless steel with particular visco-elastic properties was chosen to make initial prototypes.

Coronary artery studies in dogs established the reliability of the device for percutaneous placement [1] and determined long-term information on stent integrity in the coronary artery. Studies in artherosclerotic rabbit iliac arteries demonstrated potentially positive effects of the stents in diseased vessels, including opening of dissections caused by balloon dilatation of artherosclerotic plaques [2]. Other studies defined the histologic response in various animal models [3–5].

Clinical investigations began in 1988 with placement of the stent in cases of acute closure that required emergency bypass graft surgery. The stent was intended as a "bridge to surgery" in these patients and proved successful in

[1] Interventional Cardiology, University of Alabama at Birmingham, University Station, Birmingham, AL 35295, USA
[2] Interventional Cardiology, St. Vincents Hospital, Indiana Heart Institute Indianapolis, IN, USA

Coronary Stents
Edited by U. Sigwart and G.I. Frank
© Springer-Verlag Berlin Heidelberg 1992

establishing antegrade blood flow and clinical stability for the majority of patients as they were prepared for emergent or urgent CABG. In those patient having repeat angiography prior to discharge, the stented segment was occluded in approximately two-thirds. This observation represented our first indication of the importance of continued antiplatelet therapy and anticoagulation in maintaining good flow through the stented vessels.

Neither was possible immediately after CABG [6]. Initial clinical investigations progressed rapidly to use of the stent for definitive management of acute closure or threatened closure without CABG. Multicenter investigations began in the fall of 1989 at which time the FDA also approved investigation of the device as a primary adjunct to PTCA for treatment of restenosis.

Design and Mechanism of Action

The stent itself consists of a single strand of monofilamentous stainless steel surgical suture wire 0.006'' (0.15 mm) in diameter (Fig. 1). Newer prototypes are made from tantalum. Tantalum has two distinct advantages over stainless steel. In vitro evidence suggests the external tantalum oxide layer present on these wires is significantly more "biostable" than stainless steel

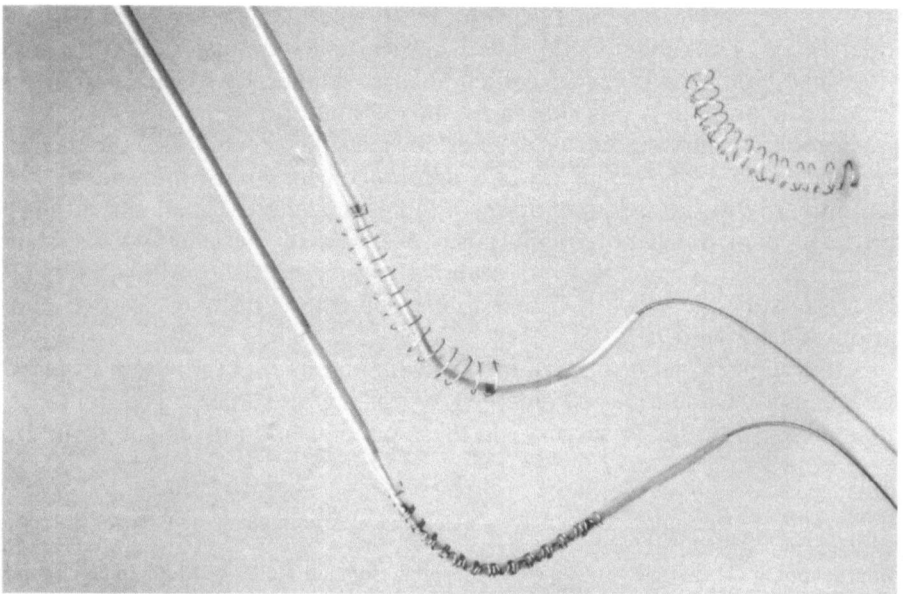

Fig. 1. Flexible balloon mounted coil before and after expansion and after balloon removal

counterparts. This may translate into a less thrombogenic device. Tantalum also is more radio-opaque which should enhance ease and accuracy of placement. This may become more important as shorter prototypes, with less overall metal are used to more precisely target focal areas of intimal tearing or vessel recoil.

The single strand of wire is carefully tooled into an incomplete "serpentine" coil which is then hand wrapped by the manufacturer (Cook Inc., Bloomington, In) onto a standard polyvinyl chloride coronary angioplasty balloon catheter (Cook). To accommodate the tightly wrapped coil, the balloon requires certain "bulk." This feature has allowed safe deployment without dislodgement of the stent but has compromised profile and trackability. The shaft is relatively stiff to enhance pushability. Because the coil design undergoes a 15%–20% recoil in diameter after expansion, it has been mounted on PVC balloons 0.5 mm in diameter bigger than the dilated size of the stent. For example, a 3.0 stent is mounted on a 3.5 balloon which

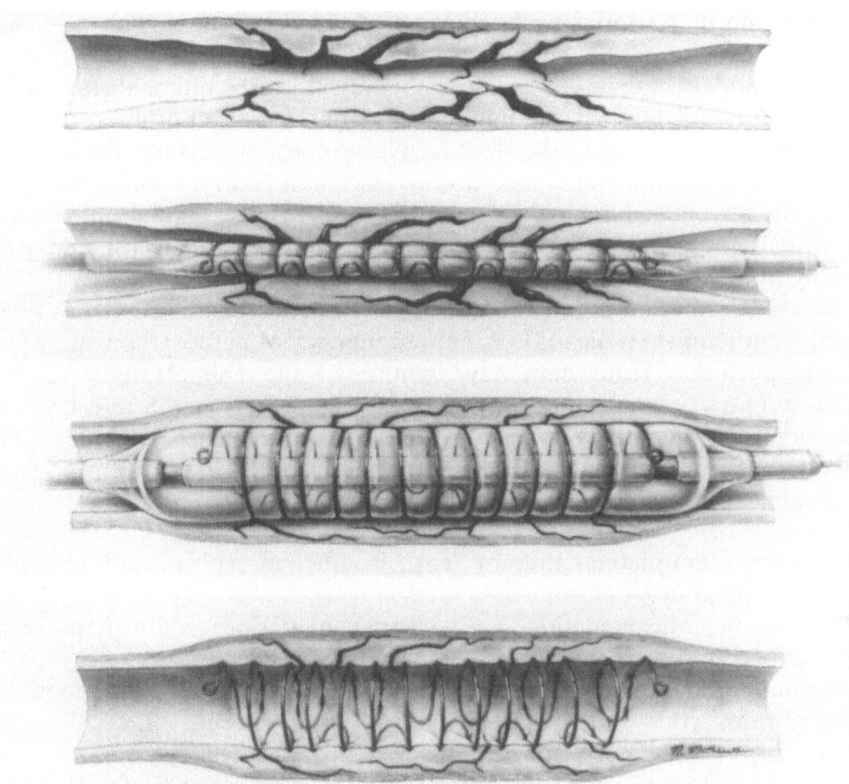

Fig. 2. Diagnostic representation of the "scaffolding" effect of the balloon-expandable coil

reaches nominal size at 6 atm of pressure. This inflation pressure is also required to fully expand the stent wires.

The coil has sufficient "plastic properties" to allow additional expansion, if necessary.

The stainless steel stents, which are difficult to visualize using standard fluoroscopy, are positioned using the proximal and distal balloon markers on the catheter. The device currently is produced in 20 mm lengths, but 12 mm and 25 mm prototypes will soon be available. The 20 mm stents are mounted on a 25 mm balloon. The stent does not shorten during expansion, and precise placement using the balloon markers is not difficult.

After expansion, the coils produce a simple circular scaffolding for the arterial lumen. Wires are approximately 1–2 mm apart and initially produce a slightly "scalloped" effect (Fig. 2). Since intimal tears and dissections are invariably longitudinal, lumenal patency is enhanced. Very rarely some material has been noted to prolapse between the wires. Additional balloon dilation usually solves the problem. Rarely a stent has been placed within a stent to enhance initial results.

Segments of atherosclerotic plaque are "stented" externally. When applied to normal arterial wall segments, the wires form shallow trenches forcing the internal elastic lamina into the media. An important observation in animal models is that 1:1 sizing in the vessel causes minor distortion of the internal elastic luminal and minimal smooth muscle cell proliferation [7]. Alternatively, oversizing of the stent or over expansion fractures the internal elastic luminal and medial layers in the vessel wall and may lodge the stent against the adventia. Under these circumstances profuse, exuberant smooth muscle cell proliferation can be induced in animal models [8] and presumably in man.

Much information about the biological response to this stent has been gained from animal studies [5]. A limited number of autopsy and surgically excised specimens from man have confirmed the animal study results. Within minutes or hours the stent wires become covered by a thin layer of fibrinogen and platelets (Fig. 3). A variety of factors which are still poorly understood limit this process in the large majority of cases. Factors which are thought to promote stent thrombosis are:

1. Inadequate antiplatelet therapy, e.g., insufficient aspirin, dipyridamole, and i.v. dextran
2. Inadequate anticoagulation, e.g., insufficient periprocedural heparin or postprocedural warfarin
3. Amount of underlying vessel wall damage, e.g., length and depth of arterial dissection
4. Presence of thrombus at dilatation site before or after dilatation
5. Poor flow characteristics of vessel, e.g., stent diameter/vessel diameter mismatch, distal dissection, distal or proximal spasm, vessel supplying nonviable myocardium, small stent/vessel size

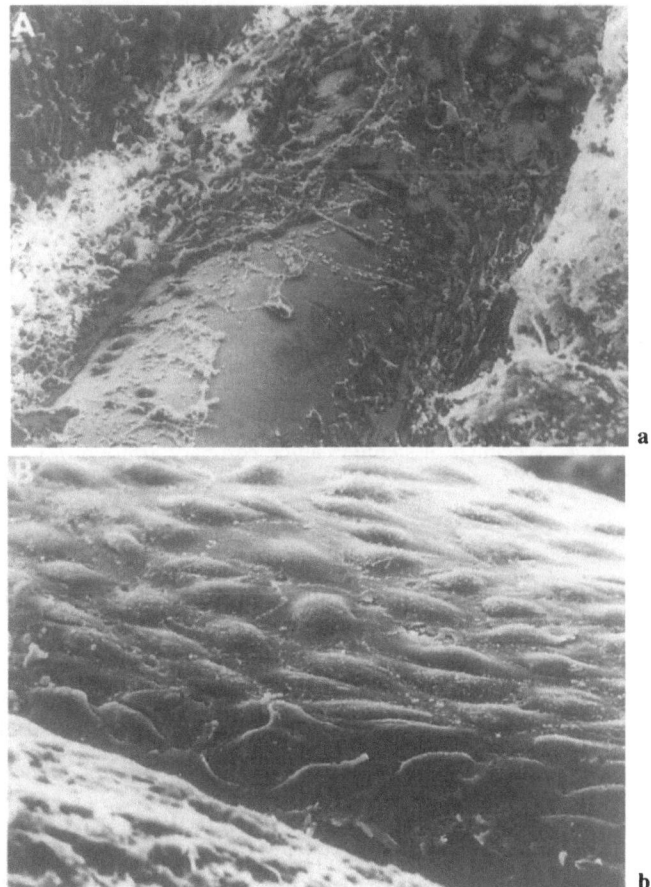

Fig. 3. a Photoelectron micrograph of stent 48 h after placement in a normal canine coronary artery. Note the fibrin, platelets, and red blood cells on the surface. **b** Stent wire at 2 weeks covered by a monolayer of endothelial cells

After 3 or 4 days, endothelial cells and smooth muscle cells are seen migrating over the stent wires. A complete lining of cells has paved the stent wires and damaged arterial surface by 14 days. The internal layer of the vessel then undergoes a period of autoregulated remodelling to produce a smooth "non-scalloped" luminal surface. "Bumps" and "trenches" produced by the stent are filled in by smooth vessel cells and their secreted polyglycan intracellular matrix (Fig. 4). Shear stress forces modulated through endothelial cell release of mitogens and antimitogenic heparin sulphates are thought to control the process. At 1–2 months, the stent is covered by a smooth layer of neointimal tissue covered by flow-directed, normal-appearing, endothelial cells. In animals not exposed to oversized

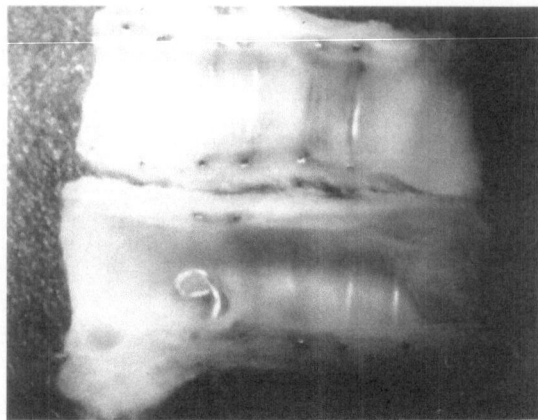

Fig. 4. Specimen of stented canine coronary artery at 6 months; note normal-appearing thin layer of neointima

stents, the neoendothelial layer is 200–400 µm in thickness and decreases over time. In patients the proliferative response is variable depending on factors not yet well understood and appears to have a 4–6 month time course of clinical/angiographic presentation not dissimilar to that seen after standard PTCA. In some patients, early restenosis has the irregular angiographic appearance of organized areas of thrombus and responds to very low repeat dilatation pressures.

Other early histological observations include focal areas of medical necrosis below the stent wires and the occasional clumping of inflammatory cells. Animals studies in dogs have been extended beyond 2 years with no unusual histological findings noted. Clinical studies thus far have confirmed the medium term, benign stability, and biocompatibility of the device in the coronary artery wall.

Current Clinical Indications and Results

Clinical indications for the use of this device are still evolving. Recommendations will change as the device itself is improved, medical management of patients receiving stents is optimized, and results of ongoing observational and randomized studies become available.

The indications for any medical procedure depend upon an analysis of the risk/benefit ratio for the individual patient concerned. Acute vessel closure and late restenosis are two entirely different problems faced by the patient having PTCA and deserve separate consideration.

Acute Closure

Acute closure during or soon after PTCA is a heterogeneous syndrome which accounts for the vast majority of the ischemic complications of PTCA. In descending order of severity these include death, Q wave myocardial infarction, emergent bypass surgery, non-Q wave myocardial infarction, and emergent repeat PTCA [5–9]. Many episodes of acute closure can be effectively managed by repeat dilatation but residual dissection is frequently present. Prolonged heparinization is usually required and some myocardial necrosis is common as is recurrent angina and lesion restenosis. The decision to attempt continued medical management in the event of an initially unsatisfactory dilatation may result in infarction or death, particularly in patients with more severe or multivessel disease. The precise incidence of these adverse outcomes has not been studied satisfactorily, because patients with these complications are usually referred for urgent or emergent CABG.

The results of emergent CABG have been better documented. The mortality ranges from 2% to 25%, depending on the center and definition of "emergent" [10, 14, 16, 17]. Significant myocardial necrosis occurs in 50%, and Q wave myocardial infarction occurs in between 25% and 60% [14, 18–25]. Emergent CABG is also associated with increased noncardiac morbidity including reoperation for rebleeding and mediastinitis, markedly increased hospital stay and costs, and the use of saphenous vein conduits as opposed to internal mammary artery grafts. This latter disadvantage to the patient is of considerable importance since the long-term patency of vein grafts is limited. Late survival is also significantly worse in patients who have a Q wave myocardial infarction complicating emergency CABG.

The benefits and risks of using the stent to treat acute closure or threatened impending closure can only be discussed against the background of knowledge of the "natural history" of acute closure. The stent has been used in approximately 200 patients (as of September 1990) with arterial dissection or acute closure. The device was successfully placed in 95% (including all cases in our series). There is a learning curve in the use of the device and particularly for placement in proximal lesions. Experienced operators are successful in better than 98% of cases. The device produces a superior or markedly improved luminal appearance in 95% of the cases (Fig. 5). There have been five device failures. In one case, the stent "accordioned" probably from failure of the operator to adequately dilate the proximal part of the vessel through which the stent had to "track". In the few cases when flow was not improved, the patient was either in full cardiac arrest at the time of stenting, or long dissections were not adequately covered by the stent, or the vessel contained large amounts of thrombus, and anticoagulation therapy had not been optimized prior to stent placement.

Of this total population with acute or threatened closure, CABG was required in 6%, and Q wave myocardial infarction occurred in 8% in spite

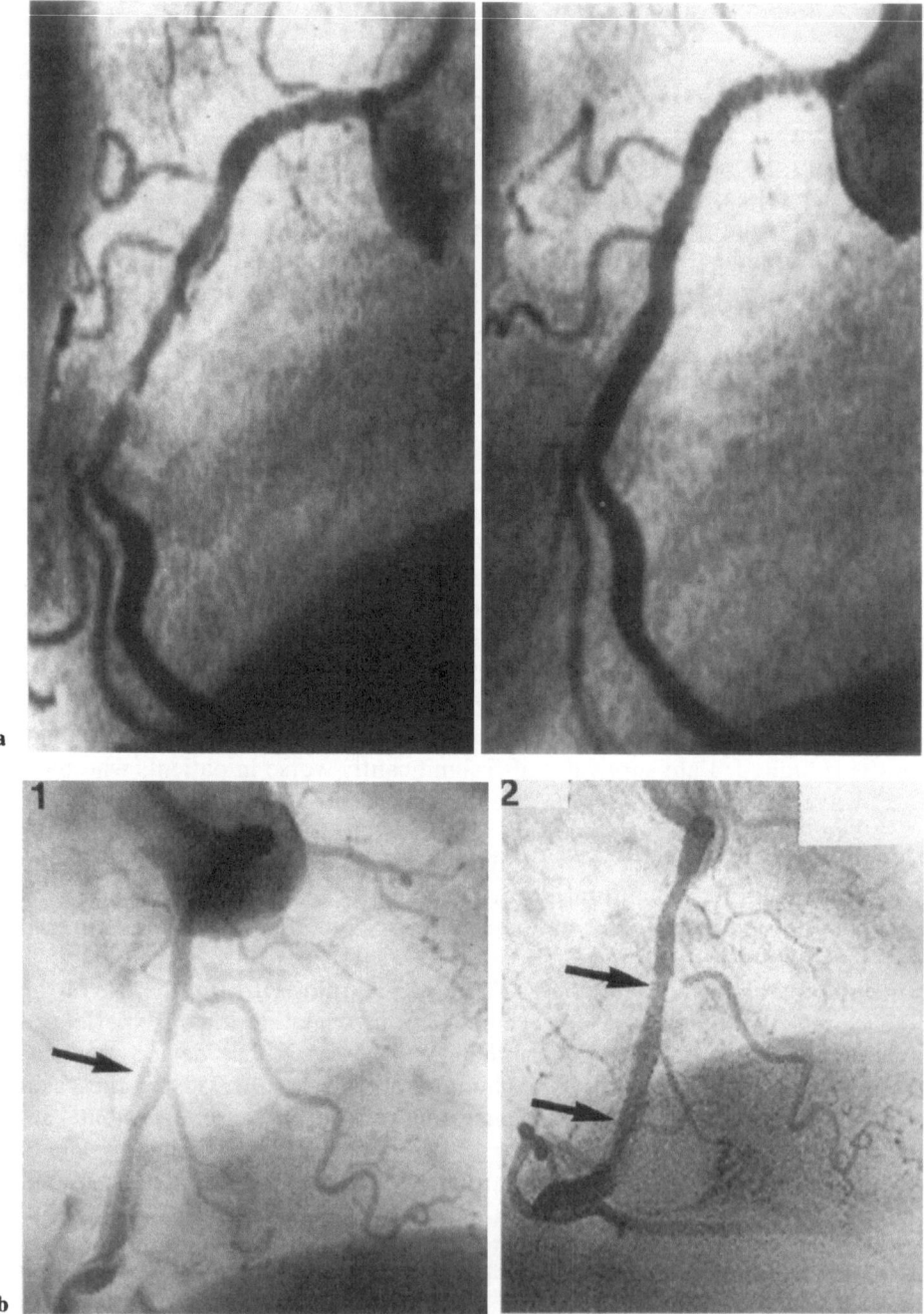

Fig. 5a,b. Dissected right coronary arteries repaired with the use of $2 \times 30\,\text{mm}$ stents

of stenting. Mortality was 1%. Whether these results are superior to what might have been expected without stenting is difficult to determine, but the incidence of CABG and Q wave MI appears to have been reduced. Acute or subacute thrombosis occurred in 6% of patients because of the reasons previously outlined. In addition, 15% of patients suffered significant bleeding complications usually from the femoral artery puncture site. Both stent thrombosis and bleeding complications have been markedly reduced in the latter part of the series. The medical management changes which have enhanced these results will be discussed later. Lesion recurrence of the stenting for dissection or acute closure occurs in up to 50% of patients within 4–6 months but is amenable to routine repeat PTCA [26].

Restenosis

Restenosis after PTCA is an important clinical problem in 25%–35% of patients, but repeat dilatation is successful in more than 95% and is complication-free in 98% [27]. Good long-term results are achieved in one-half to two-thirds of patients depending on the site of the lesion. For stenting to be used as a treatment for restenosis, the risk-benefit ratio must be superior to repeat balloon dilatation or, where appropriate, alternative therapies such as bypass surgery.

The risk from PTCA or stenting in restenotic lesions depends upon the risk profile of the patient and the nature of the lesion. Because of the utility of this device for tortuous and distal vessels, long lesions, ostial sites, and

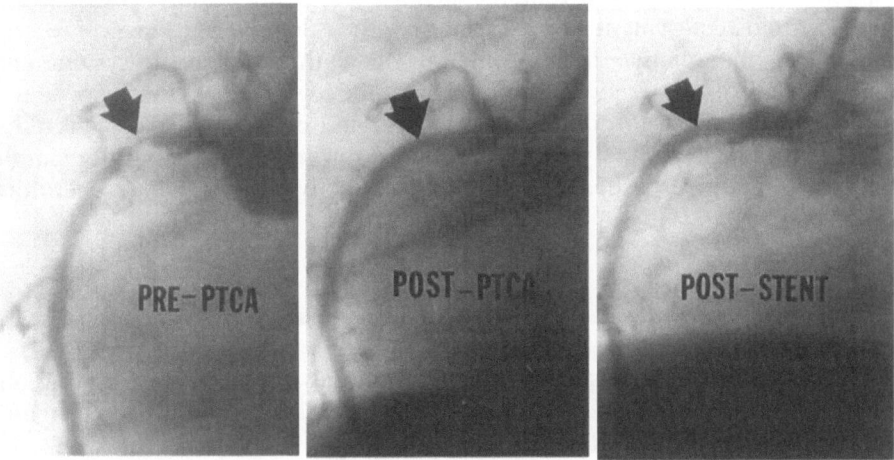

Fig. 6. From left to right, pre and post standard PTCA and after stenting. Note the improvement in luminal results after stenting. At 6 months, this patient remains free of restenosis

bypass grafts, it has been used in a heterogeneous population of patients and vessel sites with restenosis. Results have to be interpreted taking these factors into account. The device has been successfully placed in 97% of attempts. Acute or subacute thrombosis occurred in 2%, CABG was needed in 4%, and mortality has been 1%. These results also represent learning curve experience. Angiographic follow-up is incomplete at the time of writing this chapter, but to date more than 30% of patients have had angiographic restenosis (>50% diameter narrowing). Whether this represents any improvement on what might have been expected in this population with balloon dilatation alone cannot be determined, but it should be clear that stenting with this device will not solve restenosis. On theoretical grounds, stents might reduce restenosis by optimizing the initial luminal results. Since vessel wall and/or plaque recoil is probably responsible for restenosis in only 30%–40% of cases [28–30], stenting might at least be able to reduce the restenosis rate by this amount (Fig. 6). Thus, restenosis observed to date may still represent a relative improvement on what might have been otherwise achieved with balloon dilatation alone. Randomized trials will help define the role of stents for restenosis and further analysis will be required to determine which subsets of patients and lesions will benefit. Studies are needed to determine if lesions undergoing vessel wall recoil hours or days after dilatation can be identified at the time of PTCA [30].

Delivery and Deployment

From a technical perspective, deployment of this stent utilizes routine angioplasty equipment but requires advanced operator expertise. Successful delivery and deployment are associated with a definite learning curve secondary to the relative high profile of the catheter delivery system and delicate nature of the stent mounted balloon segment. Certain procedural aspects in reference to equipment selection and delivery mechanics require elaboration. The stented vessel is also more thrombogenic than after simple balloon dilatation. Critical attention to adjunctive medication is therefore required.

Preparing the Patient and Adjunctive Medical Therapy

Strict anticoagulation requirements are essential for successful stenting. In principle, high serum levels of antiplatelet agents and modest anticoagulation appears to provide the best results.

In patients undergoing elective stenting for restenosis or with lesion at high risk for dissection, aggressive pre-PTCA therapy is possible. This will include at least 2 doses of soluble aspirin 325 mg and 2 doses of dipyridamole 75 mg. Importantly, enteric-coated aspirin has proved ineffective in reliably inhibiting stent thrombosis. Calcium antagonists should also be administered and in patients with a history of peptic ulceration H_2 receptor antagonists are helpful in ensuring compliance with aspirin therapy. Dextran 40 should be administered at a dose of 75 cc/h for at least 2 h prior to PTCA. To shorten hospitalization, warfarin may be administered the day before the procedure. At angioplasty centers where stents are available, it is arguable that as a minimum all patients should be treated with aspirin and dipyridamole prior to PTCA.

In patients with acute closure or arterial dissection, dextran infusions should be instigated immediately, and the physician should check to see if adequate antiplatelet therapy was administered prior to PTCA. If not, aspirin and dipyridamole should be given in the catheterization suite. Facilities for monitoring the activated clotting time (ACT) should be available in the catheterization suite and nursing unit. During the procedure, sufficient heparin should be administered to prolong the ACT to >300 s. Stent placement should also be associated with pre- and posttreatment of the vessel with 200 mg of intracoronary nitroglycerin. If thrombus appears to be present in the stented segment after treatment, urokinase 250 000–750 000 IU should be given by slow intracoronary injection. Under special circumstances, e.g., acute myocardial infarction or thrombotic vein grafts, prolonged urokinase infusion at 80 000 IU/h for 12–18 h has proven effective.

Post Stenting. Maintenance of a strict protocol has proved very effective in minimizing complications. Sheaths should be removed 4–6 h after the procedure. Bed rest for at least 48 h has markedly reduced the incidence of groin complications. Careful initial puncture of the femoral artery below the inguinal ligament has also reduced groin complications. Excessive anticoagulation also has increased bleeding complications. It is important to critically control the anticoagulation level between narrow parameters (PTT 45–80). Patients must be managed in specialized untis where medical and nursing surveillance is optimal. The following regimen is recommended:

Prior to Sheath Removal:
1. Draw ACT every 30 min until level is <150 s
2. Remove femoral sheath when ACT < 150 s (approx. 3–4 h poststenting)
3. Continue dextran 40 infusion at 50–75 cc/h until after sheaths are removed and PTT meets criteria specified below
4. Draw PTT just prior to sheath removal:
    If PTT > 60 or <90 s, maintain groin pressure for a minimum of 45 min
    If PTT > 90 s, maintain groin pressure for a minimum of 60 min

Post Sheath Removal:
1. Draw ACT at 1 h post sheath removal and administer heparin drip (with additional boluses if necessary) to adjust ACT to approximately 200 s and/or

2. One hour post sheath removal, administer the following heparin dosage:

    If PTT > 80 s, start heparin drip at 1000 units/h

    If PTT > 65 or <79 s, give heparin bolus of 1000 units then begin heparin drip at 1000 units/h

    If PTT < 64 s, administer heparin bolus of 2000 units then begin heparin at 1000 units/h

3. Document groin checks every 30 min 4 times after heparin drip is started

4. Continue to check PTT every 6 h until heparin drip is discontinued. Maintain PTT at 45–80 s

5. Adjust the heparin treatment using the following scale:

    If PTT > 40 or <45 s, increase drip rate by 200 units/h

    If PTT > 35 or <39 s, increase drip rate by 200 units/h and give 1000 units heparin i.v. bolus

    If PTT < 34 s, increase drip rate by 200 units/h and give 2000 units heparin i.v. bolus

6. Begin the following drug regime as soon as patient can tolerate it: soluble aspirin 325 mg once a day with meals, dipyridamole 75 mg TID with meals, diltiazem 60 mg TID with meals, warfarin as needed

7. Wean patient from haparin after 3–4 days when PTT indicates adequate anticoagulation with warfarin (18–20 s). *Note*: To minimize groin bleeding complications, maintain bed rest for 36–48 h after sheath removal.

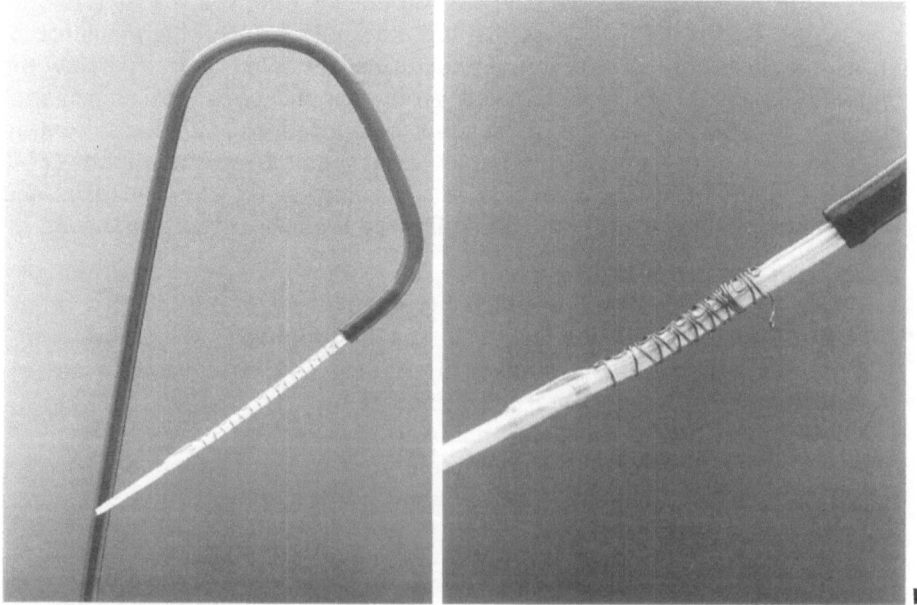

a   b

Fig. 7. a Undepolyed stent, **b** accordion effect when advancing through inadequately dilated segments

The patient discharge medication regime consists of soluble aspirin 325 mg daily, dipyridamole 75 mg TID, calcium channel agent of choice (e.g., dilitazem 60 mg QID), and warfarin for 2 months (recommended).

Lesion/Vessel Preparation

The target lesion and vessel must be adequately predilated prior to attempted stent placement. Dilatation with a balloon diameter in ratio of 1:1 with the vessel diameter is essential. Underdilatation is usually insufficient to allow passage of the stent.

Predilatation of the vessel must take into account atherosclerotic plaque proximal and distal to the lesion. Borderline obstructions may inhibit advancement of the device across the primary lesion. Excessive force applied through resistant vessel segments may result in an accordion effect on the stent (Fig. 7).

Guiding Catheter and Guidewire Selection

The flexibility of the stent design allows it to be used with standard Judkins and Amplatz catheter configurations. Care must be taken on ensure that the inside lumen of the guiding catheter is of sufficient size to allow unobstructed passage of the stent/balloon system. In general, all 8 French large lumen guideing catheters are suitable for placement of 2.0–3.0 mm devices. Large lumen 9F guiding catheters are required for the placement of 3.5 and 4.0 mm stents. Selected guiding catheters must provide excellent "backup" support for successful stent delivery. Before starting a PTCA on a complex lesion, it is worthwhile to consider the equipment which might be needed should the lesion dissect or acutely close. For example, if one is dilating a 3.5 mm vessel it might be prudent to start the case with a large lumen 9F guiding catheter and an 0.018 guidewire compatible balloon system.

In practice, the following steps can be followed. Should the lesion dissect or otherwise look unsatisfactory after adequate dilatation, the balloon is placed distal to the lesion and the initial coronary guidewire can be replaced by an "extra support" 0.018 wire. This wire is then extended and the PTCA balloon is exchanged for a "stent balloon". This maneuver can be completed rapidly if initial equipment is chosen with the stenting contingency in mind.

Successful use of the stent is enhanced with the use of 0.016 or 0.018" (0.41 or 0.46 mm) guidewires. One wire, 0.018 "Xtra Support" (ACS, Santa Clara, CA), has proved to be particularly useful. The increased size and shaft support of the 0.018 inch wires allows for vessel straightening to improve tracking through even severely tortuous vessels (Fig. 8). Distal placement of the wire is critical to position the stiff shaft of the wire within the lesion to improve crossing potential.

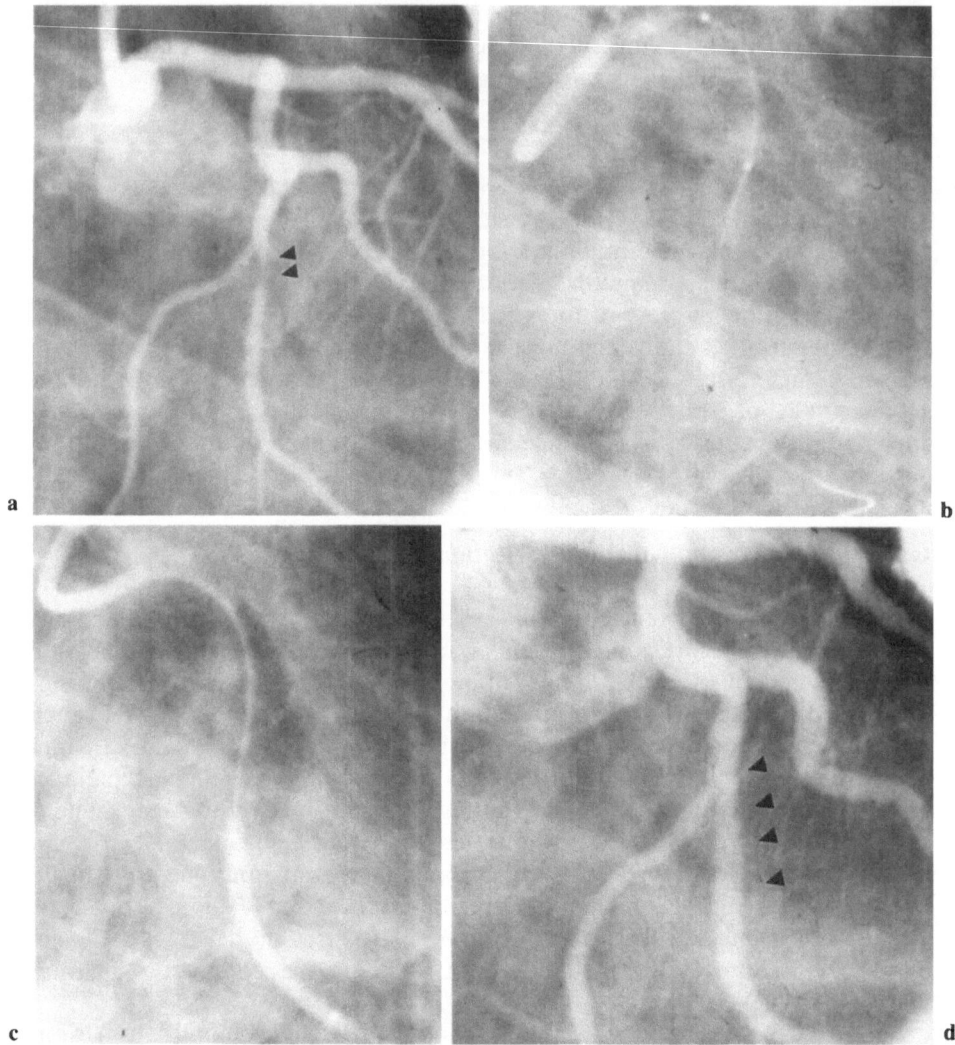

Fig. 8. a Restenosis lesion, obtuse marginal; note long left main with right angle left circumflex; **b** advancement of stent balloon around angled circumflex origin; note guide catheter position; **c** stent deployment; **d** post stent placement

Positioning and Deployment

Coaxial guide catheter positioning to the stented vessel is imperative. The stent should be advanced to the primary curve of the guiding catheter but not forwarded to the vessel until the guiding catheter has been intubated to a strong position within the ostium of the vessel. After guiding catheter

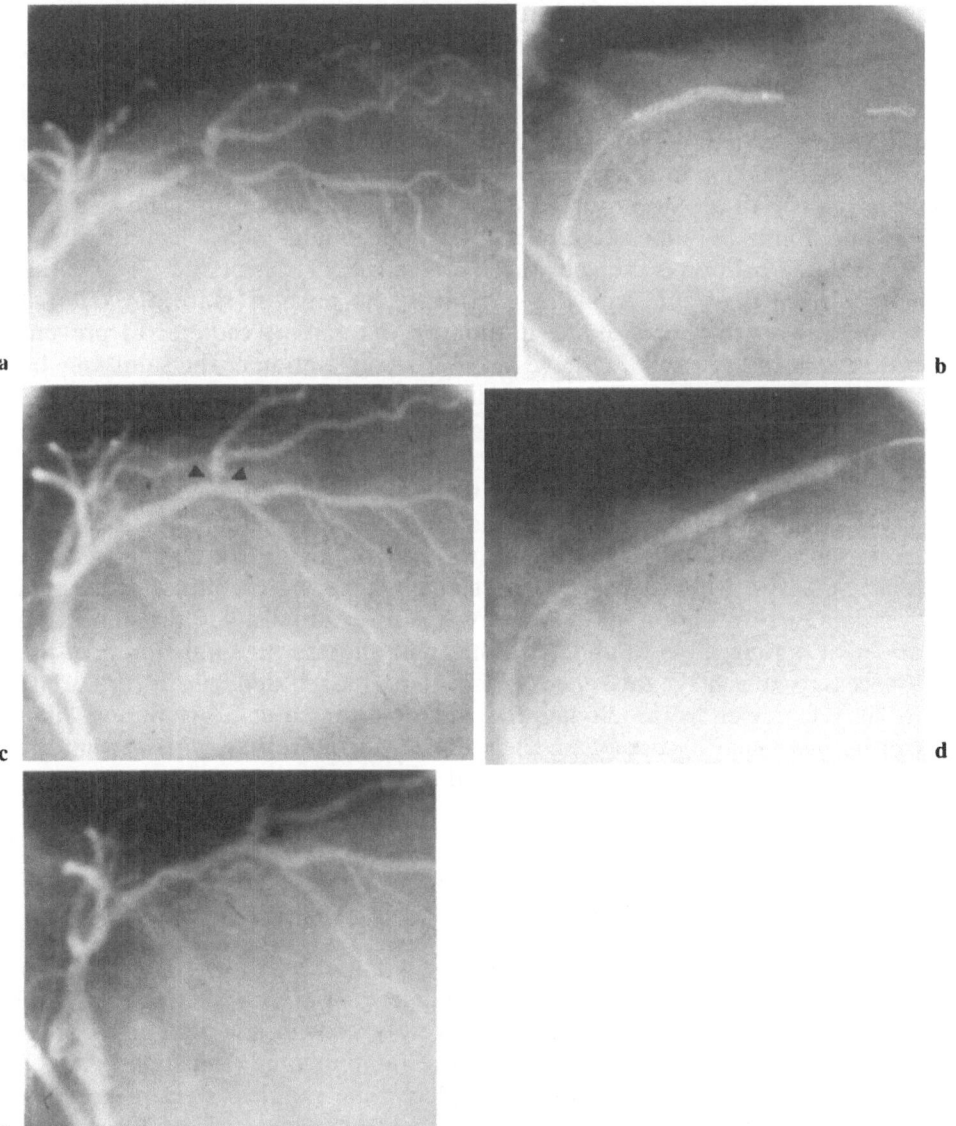

Fig. 9. a Restenosis of segmental left anterior descending artery (LAD) lesion, note diagonal lesion; **b** deployment of 2.0-mm spiral coil stent; **c** post stent placement, note stenosis at diagonal origin (*arrows*); **d** 2.0-mm balloon inflated through stent coils in diagonal origin; **e** post stent placement and PTCA of diagonal, note diagonal origin (*arrows*)

stability has been ensured, the stent is positioned across the lesion utilizing the proximal and distal markers on the balloon as a reference points. The stent begins 1–2 mm distal to the proximal marker. The proximal margin of the stent should be positioned 4–5 mm proximal to the region of the vessel to be stented. Stent deployment occurs between 4 and 6–8 atm. The inflation pressure should be increased to 6–8 atm to further compress the coils into the arterial wall and to ensure dislodgement of the stent from the balloon. The initial inflation time should be 90–120 s depending on clinical tolerance. The deflated balloon is then advanced 1–2 mm to disengage the wings of the balloon from the stent. Applying continuous negative pressure, the balloon is withdrawn while maintaining tension on the guiding catheter to prevent entrapment of the guide in the vessel. Further dilatation of the stent may be necessary with a standard, noncompliant, low profile balloon system if the angiographic result is not adequate. Branch vessels may also be accessed through the spiral coil if necessary (Fig. 9). If angiographic evidence of thrombus is present, intracoronary lytic therapy may be utilized.

It is important to remember that the delivery balloon has a 0.5 mm larger diameter than the stent. Since the balloon material is compliant, care must be taken when deploying the stent in tapering or diffusely diseased vessels. Over-distension may cause arterial dissection distal to the stent. If in doubt, it is preferable to undersize the stent and use high inflation pressure if necessary to achieve the required size. In part, each stent can be "tailored" to fit the vessel by modifying the inflation pressures. A tapering stent can be fashioned by deploying the stent at 5–6 atm, then withdrawing the balloon half-way through the stent, and again inflating to 8 atm.

Future Developments

Currently, tantalum prototypes of varying lengths are completing successful investigations in animal models as are prototypes with a variety of polymer-pharmacologic coatings. Tantalum is more radio-opaque than stainless steel, and tantalum stents will be easier to place than stainless steel prototypes. More importantly, visibility will enable the stent to be removed if necessary should the stent be misplaced. Fine "biopsy-like" forceps can be used to remove the stent in the form of a single strand of fine wire. Such maneuvers have been performed in animal models. Tantalum may have other advantages. There is a body of data which suggests tantalum may be less thrombogenic and more "biostable" than stainless steel. Tantalum also has different visco-elastic properties and may be less likely to fracture the internal elastic lumina on expansion. Since fracture of the internal elastic lumina and damage to smooth muscle cells probably increases the degree of neointimal proliferation, this may prove to be an advantage.

Stainless steel is, however, more cosmetically pleasing since it is almost invisible within the vessel. The current coil stents have now been in place in some patients for 3 years and other stent designs for over 5 years. Now with some thousands of stainless steel devices in place, there has been a remarkable lack of any long-term problems related to biostability. There have been no incidents of infection, migration, fracture, perforation, or late allergenic or other problems. It seems that after the first 4–6 months, this family of stainless steel devices becomes an invisible and benign part of the vessel wall. Tantalum is expected to produce similar if not superior long-term results, but its presence will be apparent. The amount of metal visible will be a minute fraction of that which remains in the chest after bypass graft surgery. Bioabsorbable polymer alterations of the current designs are under review, but given the physical disadvantages of polymers in the single-strand coil format, there seems to be little advantage to the bioabsorbable properties.

Polymers do facilitate the bonding of pharmacologic agents. To this end, a thin layer of polymer has been successfully coated on both stainless steel and tantalum coil stents. A variety of pharmacologic agents have been incorporated in these polymers utilizing established sustained release drug technology. Animal models are currently being used to investigate the potential of these approaches. For example, a polymer-heparin prototype has been successfully implanted in the carotid arteries of swine without adjunctive systemic anticoagulation [7]. Other studies involve the use of hirudin, a potent antithrombin agent. Antimitotic-antiproliferative agents are also under investigation. There is much work to be done in this area, but potential value exists for stents as delivery devices for locally targeted pharmacological therapy.

Simple changes in stent design soon to be investigated clinically may also improve results. Shorter 12-mm stents should be more trackable and easier to insert. Since they contain 40% less metal, they should be less thrombogenic. For long dissections, a 25-mm prototype has been developed in an attempt to avoid the need for placing tandem stents. The availability of stents of varying lengths may provide the operation with greater flexibility in optimizing luminal results.

The current delivery balloon is also undergoing improvements which could improve the ease of stent delivery.

Conclusions

This stent has demonstrated the capacity to reliably "scaffold" dissected vessels (Fig. 10) or arterial segments undergoing acute recoil or collapse. To what extent this will improve the safety and efficacy of balloon dilatation remains to be determined. Early results, however, suggest the need for

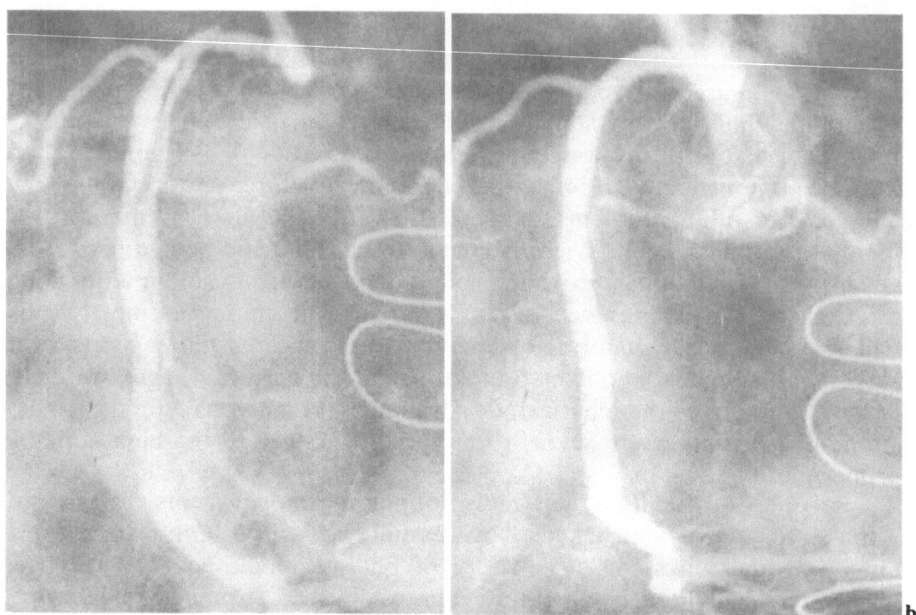

a   b

Fig. 10a,b. Right coronary artery with severe spiral dissection before and after stenting

emergency surgery can be almost eliminated once experience is gained with effective deployment of the device. It also appears that thrombosis and bleeding complications can be minimized to acceptable levels once the angioplasty team has mastered the simple but critical nursing and medical management skills required for the stent patient. In some respects, the difficulty with stenting begins after the patient leaves the angioplasty suite. The factors that need reemphasizing are conservative but well-monitored anticoagulation and cautious ambulation. The current development of "vascular plug" devices and methods for the femoral artery may facilitate more rapid ambulation in the future. The current need for prolonged hospitalization to stabilize anticoagulation may be obviated in the future by prehospitalization therapy with warfarin in combination with local femoral artery vascular hemostasis techniques. This will markedly reduce the cost of hospitalization for stented patients.

The question of cost, however, requires additional consideration. Although the cost of PTCA plus stent for acute closure is increased, it is still markedly less than would be incurred if the patient required emergency bypass surgery. If the stent is used electively to prevent restenosis, however, the equation changes, unless stenting is used as an alternative to bypass surgery and/or has a high degree of long-term success.

Most importantly, successful stent technology will add a certain predictability to the technique of balloon dilatation. This should apply to "ideal" lesions as well as long, tortuous, and complex lesions not otherwise suitable for percutaneous revascularization. Stenting should prevent CABG and Q-wave myocardial infarction in patients at risk of acute closure. Mortality may also be reduced. Angiographic restenosis at the stented vessel site can be expected in 30%–50% of cases, depending on the degree of damage to the vessel wall. The vast majority can be treated with a low-risk repeat dilatation and a 2-day (one night) hospital stay. Many asymptomatic patients with angiographic restenosis can be managed medically. This appears to be a reasonable compromise for avoiding emergency CABG and MI. Accordingly, in combination with enhanced balloon technology, coronary artery stenting shows considerable promise as a means of expanding the application of PTCA to lesions which woud otherwise be unapproachable. This may be most important in the use of PTCA in extensive multivessel coronary artery disease.

References

1. Roubin GS, Robinson KA, King SB III, Gianturco C, Black AJ, Brown JE, Siegel RJ, Douglas JS Jr (1987) Early and late results of intracoronary arterial stenting after coronary angioplasty in dogs. Circulation 76(4):891–897
2. Robinson KA, Roubin GS, Siegel RJ, Black AJ, Apkarian RP, King SB III (1988) Intra-arterial stenting in the atherosclerotic rabbit. Circulation 78(3):646–653
3. Robinson KA, Roubin GS, King SB, Siegel R, Rodgers G, Apkarian RP (1989) Correlated microscopic observations of arterial responses to intravascular stenting. Scan Micro 3(2):665–679
4. Rodgers GP, Minor ST, Robinson K, Cromeens D, Woolbert SC, Stephens LC, Guyton JR, Wright K, Roubin GS, Raizner AE (1990) Adjuvant therapy for intracoronary stents (investigations in atherosclerotic swine). Circulation 82(2):560–569
5. Garratt KN, Heras M, Holmes DR Jr, Roubin GS, Chesebro JH (1990) Platelet deposition and thrombosis in arterial stents: effect of hirudin compared with heparin plus antiplatelet therapy. J Am Coll Cardiol 15(11):109A
6. Roubin GS, Douglas JS Jr, Lembo NJ, Black AJ, King SB III (1988) Intracoronary stenting for acute closure following percutaneous transluminal coronary angioplasty (PTCA). Circulation 78(II):407
7. Cavender JB, Anderson P, Roubin GS (1990) The effects of heparin bonded tantalum stents on thrombosis and neointimal proliferation. Circulation 82(4) [Suppl III]:541
8. Schwartz RS, Murphy JG, Edwards WD, Camrud AR, Vlietstra RE, Holmes DR (1990) Restenosis occurs with internal elastic lamina laceration and is proportional to severity of vessel injury in a porcine coronary artery model. Circulation 82(4) [Suppl III]:656
9. Roubin G, Talley J, Anderson H, Murphy D, Guyton R, Jones E, Craver J, Lembo N, Douglas J, King S (1987) Morbidity and mortality associated with emergency bypass graft surgery following elective coronary angioplasty. J Am Coll Cardiol 9:11–124A
10. Anderson H, Cox W, Roubin G, Weintraub W, Douglas J, King S (1987) Mortality of acute closure following coronary angioplasty (PTCA). J Am Coll Cardiol 9:II-20A
11. Bredlau CE, Roubin GS, Leimgruber PP, Douglas JS Jr, King SB III, Gruentzig AR (1985) In-hospital morbidity and mortality inpatients undergoing elective coronary angioplasty. Circulation 72(5):1044–1052

12. Ellis SG, Roubin GS, King SB III, Douglas JS Jr, Weintraub W, Thomas RG, Cox WR (1988) Angiographic and clinical predictors of acute closure after native vessel coronary angioplasty. Circulation 77(2):372–379
13. Detre K, Holobkov R, Kelsey S, Cowley K, Kent K, Williams D, Myler R, Faxon D, Holmes D Jr, Bounassa M, Block P, Gosselon A, Rentivoglco L, Leatherman L, Dorros G, King S, Galicia J, Al-Bassam M, Leon M, Robertson T, Passamani E (1988) Percutaneous transluminal coronary angioplasty in 1985–1986 and 1977–1981. The National Heart, Lung and Blood Institute Registry. N Engl J Med 318:265–270
14. Jacobs AK, Steenkiste A, Ruocco NA Jr, Detre KM, Ryan TJ, Faxon DP (1990) Is prior CABG a risk for angioplasty? A report from the 1985–86 NHLBI PTCA Registry. Circulation 82(4) [Suppl III]:618
15. Black AJR, Namay DC, Niederman AC, Lembo NJ, Roubin GS, Douglas JS Jr, King SB III (1989) Tear or dissection after coronary angioplasty: morphologic correlates of an ischemic complication. Circulation 79(5):1035–1042
16. Hockberg MS, Gregory JJ, McCullough J, Geilchinsky I, Houssain SM, Fuzesi L, Parsonnet V (1990) Outcome of emergent coronary artery bypass following failed angioplasty. Circulation 82 [Suppl III]:361
17. Buffet P, Villemot JP, Amrein D, Etherenot G, Juilliere E, Danchin Cherrier F (1990) Long term outcome after emergency coronary artery bypass surgery in failed angioplasty. Circulation 82 [Suppl III]:296
18. Talley JD, Weintraub WS, Rougin GS, Douglas JS Jr, Anderson HV, Jones EL, Morris DC, Liberman MA, Craver JM, Guyton RA, King SB III (1990) Failed elective percutaneous transluminal coronary angioplasty requiring coronary artery bypass surgery. Circulation 82:1203–1213
19. Reul GJ, Cooley DA, Hallman GL, Nuncan MJ, Livesay JT, Frazier HO, Ott DA, Angelini P, Massomi A, Marthur VS (1984) Coronary artery bypass for unsuccessful percutaneous transluminal coronary angioplasty. J Thorac Surg 88:685–694
20. Page VS, Ouies EJ, Colburn LQ, Bigelow JC, Saloman NW, Krause AH (1986) Percutaneous transluminal coronary angioplasty: a growing surgical problem. J Thorac Cardiovasc Surg 92:847–852
21. Golding LAR, Loop FD, Hollman JL, Franco I, Borsh J, Stewart RW, Lytle BW (1986) Early results of emergency surgery after coronary angioplasty. Circulation 74 [Suppl III]:111–126
22. Tebbe V, Roschewski W, Knake W, Herse B, Figulla HR, Klein HH, Wiegand V, Dalichan K, Kreuter H (1989) Will emergency coronary bypass grafting after failed elective percutaneous transluminal coronary angioplasty prevent myocardial infarction. Thorac Cardiovasc Surg 37:308–312
23. Murphy DA, Craver JA, Jones EL, Curling PE, Guyton RA, King SB III, Gruentzig AR, Hatcher CR JR (1984) Surgical management of acute myocardial ischemia following percutaneous transluminal coronary angioplasty. J Thorac Cardiovasc Surg 87:337–339
24. Dorros G, Conley MJ, Simpson J, Bentivoglio LG, Block P, Bourassa M, Detre K, Gosseun AJ, Gruentzig AR, Kelsey SF, Kent KM, Mock MB, Mollin SM, Myler RK, Passamani ER, Stertzer SH, Williams DO (1983) Percutaneous transluminal coronary angioplasty: report of complications from the National Heart Lung and Blood Institute PTCA Registry. Circulation 67:723–730
25. Haraphongse M, NA-Ayudhya RK, Burton J, Tymchak A, Homen D, Montaque T (1990) Clinical efficacy of emergency bypass surgery for failed coronary angioplasty. Can J Cardiol 6(5):186–190
26. Roubin GS, Hearn JA, Carlin SF, Lembo NJ, Douglas JS Jr, King SB III (1990) Angiographic and clinical follow-up in patients receiving a balloon expandable stainless steel stent (Cook, Inc.) for prevention or treatment of acute closure after PTCA. Circulation 82(4) [Suppl III]:191
27. Black AJ, Anderson HV, Roubin GS, Powelson SW, Douglas JS Jr, King SB III (1988) Repeat coronary angioplasty: correlates of a second restenosis. J Am Coll Cardiol 11(4):714–718

28. Waller BF, Pinkerton CA, Orr CM, Slack JD, VanTassel JW (1990) Circulation 82(4) [Suppl III]:314
29. Kuntz RE, Schmidt DA, Levine MJ, Reis GJ, Safian RD, Baim DS (1990) Importance of post-procedure luminal diameter on restenosis following new coronary interventions. Circulation 82(4) [Suppl III]:314
30. Lehmann KG, Feuer JM, Kumamoto KS, Le HM (1990) Elastic recoil following coronary angioplasty: magnitude and contributory factors. Circulation 82(4) [Suppl III]:313

Stenting of Coronary Arteries –
The Ideal Revascularization Technique:
Reality, Dream, Mystery or Myth?

D.P. FOLEY, H.M. VAN BEUSEKOM, B.H. STRAUSS, W.J. VAN DER GIESSEN, and P.W. SERRUYS[1]

Introduction

The late Andreas Grüntzig performed the first nonoperative dilatation of a coronary artery narrowing (or "percutaneous transluminal coronary angioplasty" – as he christened his creation), in Zurich, Switzerland, in September 1987 [1]. Happily for Dr. Grüntzig, the patient, and indeed for modern science, in particular the then burgeoning specialty of "interventional cardiology" (a term also coined by Grüntzig), the procedure was successful. Furthermore, 10 years later, that first patient underwent repeat angiography (during an "angioplasty course" at Emory University) revealing no restenosis. Percutaneous transluminal coronary angioplasty (PTCA) is now practised worldwide and offered to patients as a viable alternative to coronary artery bypass graft surgery or pharmacological therapy.

Despite its undoubted popularity and the considerable technological improvements over the years, substantial mystery still lingers, enshrouding this treatment modality. Firstly, we really do not know how it "works" or, why it "works" in some patients and not in others; secondly, we are not quite certain how to describe the impact of treatment with PTCA on the beneficiary – by the effect on the lesion itself as assessed by coronary angiography, or by the effect on coronary blood flow, which is measurable by various techniques, or by the effect on myocardial perfusion which is also objectively quantifiable, or indeed, by its impact on the wellbeing of the patient, which cannot actually be measured, but is the primary aim of the treatment as offered (since there is, as yet, no widely accepted evidence supporting a beneficial effect of PTCA on longevity, unlike CABG in certain patient subgroups). Thirdly, similar difficulties exist regarding the assessment of the long-term benefit of PTCA, which are further compounded by the variable response, over time, of the vessel wall to balloon dilatation, a process known as "restenosis". The main difficulties in this area

[1] Catheterisation Laboratory, Thoraxcenter, Erasmus University Rotterdam, P.O. Box 1738, 3000 DR Rotterdam, The Netherlands
Dr. Foley is a Research Fellow of the Irish Heart Foundation, Dr. Strauss is a Research Fellow of the Canadian Heart Foundation.

Coronary Stents
Edited by U.Sigwart and G.I. Frank
© Springer-Verlag Berlin Heidelberg 1992

are that: (a) the pathology of the process is poorly understood, and much conjecture and doubt still lingers; (b) there is no universal agreement on how to define "restenosis"; and (c) although angiography appears to be the best *widely available* descriptive technique, many investigators continue to use antiquated analysis methodology, the inaccuracy of which has been frequently and conclusively demonstrated.

Fourthly, the introduction of new devices, designed to ablate coronary artery narrowings, recanalize occluded vessels, or maintain patency by artificial endoluminal support, and thereby prevent restenosis, instead of bringing answers or solutions, has further compounded the problem, by thus far "failing to deliver the goods", while increasing the armamentarium, and therefore, "the doctor's dilemma". It is currently difficult to evaluate the relative merits of each intervention and to define their role in clinical cardiology since randomized prospective clinical trials have only recently been commenced. In applying this new technology, as with most new developments enthusiasm has been allowed to somewhat compromise objectivity, and the cardiologist has been limiting his concern to the technical and procedural aspects, while sometimes overlooking the complex biological and physiological mechanisms of atherosclerosis, and, in particular, of the restenosis process. In achieving the perceived benefit of the therapeutic intervention with these transluminal revascularization devices, the vessel wall is subjected to thermal and mechanical insults, which may have hidden long-term consequences such as the restenosis process, which has now been Iatrogenically induced in hundreds of thousands of patients.

Intravascular Stenting: Background

One of the "recent" developments has been the use of endoluminal vascular prostheses, although in fact, the original concept precedes the introduction of interventional cardiology by many decades. The intravascular stent had its first application in the animal model as early as 1912, when Carrel [2] described his experiences with "permanent intubation of the thoracic aorta", using short glass, aluminium, and gold-plated aluminium tubes in 11 dogs. He concluded that as long as no laceration of the vascular wall occurred, no thrombosis would ensue, and that improvement of the geometry and design of the tubes would prevent these problems. Unfortunately, the author had no better materials available to him and no further progress was made. In 1969 Dotter [3] published the results of his experiments with impervious plastic tube grafts in normal dog femoral and popliteal arteries, showing complete thrombosis in all cases, within 24 h [3]. There was considerable improvement in outcome when he used stainless steel coils and additional heparin for 4 days after implantation [4].

Since then, many design variations have been introduced, including: thermal shape memory alloy stents [4–7], self-expanding steel spirals [8], self-expandable stainless steel mesh stents [9–12], balloon expandable slotted stainless steel tubes [13–16], self-expanding zig-zag stents [17–19], balloon expanded U-configuration bends [20], balloon expandable inter-digitating coils [21–23], balloon expandable tantalum helical coil stents [24], balloon-expandable knitted tantalum wire stents [25, 26], removable, metallic mesh stents [27], and synthetic polymeric and biodegradable stents [28]. These various devices differ greatly in their fundamental geometry (mesh, single wire), composition (metal, plastic) and mechanical behaviour (active or passive expansion). Furthermore, there are additional subtle dif-ferences which may be important in themselves, such as thickness of filaments, alloy composition, electrostatic behaviour, and the use of biocompatible or therapeutic coatings.

More than 5 years have passed since the first clinical report of successful coronary stent implantations [9]. Although the current world experience is now in the thousands, the clinical indications and applications remain un-resolved, and even experienced investigators are still uncertain as to the ultimate role of this device in clinical cardiology. The current status of the coronary stent parallels that of the other recently introduced technological "advances" which include laser and atherectomy (directional and non-directional types). This raises a fundamental question: Have we been unable to realize the full potential of these newer devices, because of our limited understanding of the underlying biological interactions, particularly those responsible for restenosis? In this review, we will attempt to address several relevant issues based on our own experiences in the evaluation of various coronary stents and other devices for percutaneous coronary revascularization.

Clinical Application of Stenting: Simplified Stent Philosophy

There are, essentially, two undesirable consequences of PTCA for which implantation of a stent might be useful.

Abrupt Closure During or Soon After PTCA

Abrupt closure following PTCA occurs in 2%–11% of procedures [29–32]. Intimal flaps induced by the arterial injury can disrupt flow by partially or completely occluding the lumen. Sluggish antegrade flow and exposure of the media to procoagulant blood-borne elements are potent thrombogenic stimuli which further contribute to the process. The coronary stent, by acting as a splint, can physically contain the protruding obstructive flap and maintain flow, as well as possibly preventing distal embolization of macro-scopic debris originating from the plaque or flap [33]. This scaffolding function appears to be a property common to both balloon-expandable and self-expanding prostheses. Angiographic studies following stent implantation have shown that the self-expanding Wallstent and the balloon-expandable tantalum Wiktor stent both have a smoothing effect which reduces calcu-lated Poiseuille and turbulent contributions to flow resistance [11, 34]. Several reports have documented successful deployment of the various types of stents in the "bail-out" situation where the presence of intimal dissection has led to a poor result or even a life-threatening haemodynamic situation [35, 36].

Restenosis

Progressive luminal renarrowing in the months following the procedure continues to be the major limitation of coronary angioplasty. At the present time, restenosis is angiographically determined and is traditionally categorized

Table 1. A selection of criteria for angiographic restenosis in current use

Criteria	Reference
1. Loss at follow-up of at least 50% of the initial gain after PTCA (NHLBI 4)	[37]
2. A return to within 10% of the pre-PTCA diameter stenosis (NHLBI 3)	[38]
3. An immediate post-PTCA diameter stenosis <50% that increases to ≥50% at follow up	[38, 39]
4. As for 3 above, but a diameter stenosis ≥70% at follow-up (NHLBI 2)	[40]
5. Loss of ≥20% diameter stenosis from post-PTCA to follow-up	[41]
6. Loss of ≥30% diameter stenosis from post-PTCA to follow-up (NHLBI 1)	[39]
7. A diameter stenosis ≥50% at follow-up	[42]
8. A diameter stenosis ≥70% at follow-up	[43]
9. Area stenosis ≥85% at follow-up	[44]
10. Loss ≥1 mm² in stenosis area from post-PTCA to follow-up	[45]
11. Deterioration of ≥0.72 mm in minimal luminal diameter from post-PTCA to follow-up	[46]
12. Deterioration of ≥0.5 mm in minimal luminal diameter from post-PTCA to follow-up	[47]
13. Diameter stenosis >50% at follow-up of a successfully dilated lesion (defined as diameter stenosis <50%, and a gain of >10% in luminal diameter, immediately after PTCA), excluding lesions with a <10% deterioration in diameter stenosis since PTCA	[48]

NHLBI 1, 2, 3, and 4 are four different criteria for angiographic restenosis, as defined by the National Heart, Lung, and Blood Institute of the United States of America.
PTCA, percutaneous transluminal coronary angioplasty.

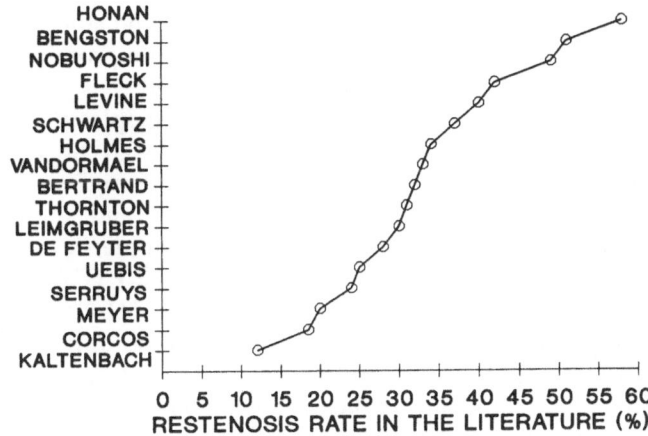

Fig. 1. Restenosis rates from a selection of published studies with different angiographic follow-up rates (57%–100%), follow-up intervals (1–9 months), 11 different restenosis criteria and various angiographic analysis techniques

according to definitions which attempt to reflect a significant deterioration in the luminal diameter of a lesion which had previously been successfully dilated. As a consequence of the lack of uniformity of definition (Table 1) [37–48], angiographic follow-up studies have documented a restenosis rate which varies between 12% and 60% (Fig. 1), in the first 6 months following PTCA. Such "definitions" cannot reflect the physiological or haemodynamic situation and, moreover, do not necessarily indicate a common underlying pathological substrate. Diverse histological processes may be responsible for restenosis, depending on the time interval since angioplasty.

Early Restenosis. Up to 11% of lesions may exhibit "restenosis" as early as 1–4 days following PTCA [49, 50]. We believe that the early cases of angiographic worsening are a result of several processes, including elastic recoil, vasospasm, sub-intimal haemorrhage or haematoma formation and/ or platelet – fibrin thrombi [50, 50a]. This time interval is too brief for significant fibrointimal hyperplasia to have occurred, for several reasons. Pathological studies of vessels which have been retrieved less than 10 days after PTCA have not shown any significant intimal hyperplasia [51–54]. Animal experiments have demonstrated that following balloon endothelial denudation in carotid arteries of rats, smooth muscle cell migration into the intima only begins at 4 days and maximal intimal smooth muscle cell proliferation is not noted before 7 days [55, 56]. Furthermore, cell cultures of medial smooth muscle cells have shown that the modulation of phenotype from the quiescent, contractile state (typical of normal medial smooth muscle cells) to a metabolically active, synthetic state only occurs after 6–7 days [57]. Smooth muscle cells obtained from intimal thickenings phenotypically resemble these synthetic-type smooth muscle cells observed in culture and share a common cytoskeleton protein profile that differs from typical medial smooth muscle cells [58, 59].

Elastic recoil following balloon angioplasty has only recently been recognized as a real phenomenon [60–65] as a result of quantitative angiographic and intravascular ultrasound studies. Rensing et al. assessed 151 coronary segments before, during, and immediately after balloon dilatation using a validated videodensitometric technique. The minimal luminal cross-section area (MLCA) before PTCA was $1.1 \pm 0.9\,mm^2$ [60]. Immediately following the procedure the MLCA of the dilated vessel was $2.8 \pm 1.4\,mm^2$. Elastic recoil, defined as the difference between the balloon MLCA ($5.2 \pm 1.6\,mm^2$) and the vessel MLCA after PTCA, was calculated to be $2.4 \pm 1.4\,mm^2$, which is almost 50% of the cross-sectional area of the fully inflated balloon. In an angiographic study of the initial 117 stent implants, we have demonstrated that the self-expanding Wallstent mitigates the effects of elastic recoil. Stenting immediately improved the MLCA from $3.0 \pm 1.2\,mm^2$ after angioplasty to $5.5 \pm 2.7\,mm^2$. In a subgroup of patients who underwent angiography 24 h later, the stent continued to expand and increased the MLCA to $6.8 \pm 4.4\,mm^2$ [66].

Late Restenosis. Two processes have been implicated in the development of late restenosis. Organization and fibrous conversion of platelet – fibrin thrombi, which can form at the site of intimal damage, may play a part; however, a more important mechanism appears to be marked cellular proliferation within the vessel wall which is precipitated by complex interactions between platelets adherent to the traumatized intima, a plethora of substances consequently released from the damaged platelets, macrophages, endothelial cells and medial smooth muscle cells, which have presumably migrated from the media into the intima, resulting in variable degrees of luminal narrowing [53, 67]. Immunoperoxidase staining of the cellular component of this fibrointimal tissue has identified the characteristic cytoskeleton proteins of medial smooth muscle cells – alpha actin, desmin and vimentin – confirming the origin of the cells responsible for this growth.

Pathology of Restenosis

Angioscopic and postmortem studies have revealed that vascular injury is frequently extensive as a consequence of PTCA, with angioscopic evidence of intimal disruption, to some extent, immediately after successful dilation, in virtually all cases, while angiography appeared normal in two thirds [68]. These findings are corroborated by autopsy findings of a high incidence of intimal dissection, haemorrhage and thrombus formation, even in the context of an angiographically successful procedure, in patients who died within 30 days of PTCA [69]. In addition, severe medial injury may be caused without angiographic abnormality [69].

Two smooth muscle cell phenotypes are distinguishable by microscopy: the synthetic, which is secretory, producing extracellular matrix proteoglycan and collagen, and appears to be responsive to growth factors [70]; and the quiescent contractile smooth muscle cell, which predominates in normal media, and has vasomotion and structural support functions. Post-mortem studies in patients who died up to several years after PTCA are (fortunately for the future of the procedure as a treatment option!) scarce and involve small patient numbers. It is, nevertheless, possible to glean that, in the majority of cases, smooth muscle cell proliferation takes place, to variable degrees, from the second week after PTCA. Findings in lesions where PTCA has been carried out more than 2 years previously appear to be histologically indistinguishable from conventional atherosclerotic plaque [54]. What happens in between these times is controversial.

In the early weeks and months after injury, synthetic type cells appear to predominate, to be gradually replaced by contractile cells. The exact temporal sequence of this phenotypic reversion is the subject of incomplete and conflicting information. Nobuyoshi's group reports predominance of synthetic cell type up to 6 months after PTCA in a post mortem study [54], whereas Strauss et al. uncovered an earlier return to the contractile state with no evidence of proliferating cells 3 months after injury, and over 70% contractile phenotype at 4 months, in tissue removed by atherectomy from stented and nonstented vessels [71]. Not unexpectedly, the extracellular matrix substance is seen to differ in accordance with the predominant cell type, with abundance of proteoglycans (chondroitin sulphate, dermatan sulphate and heparin sulphate) early, and mainly collagen later, associated with a lesser matrix volume [72].

Although cellular proliferation and matrix synthesis are recognized as the components of the restenosis lesion, the remodelling of the vessel wall after vessel injury is not understood and the relative contribution (and possibly the preeminent role) of the matrix components (proteoglycans and collagen) has not been appreciated. Since cellular proliferation appears to be an early event, the cellularity of an individual lesion is primarily related to the amount of synthesized matrix. The wide range of cell density at a particular interval in time may be related to either inherent biological variability, or, possibly, a sampling error. The total amount of matrix present at a particular time is related to the synthesis and resorption of the particular component. The turnover of proteoglycans is unknown, although the limited data indicated low collagen and elastin turnover in experimental models of hypertension [73]. The individual variability in cell density emphasizes the differential importance of matrix deposition in individual lesions. Clearly, the determination of the composition and extent of matrix synthesis, during remodelling of the vessel after injury, is a vital step in the understanding of the restenosis process and might lead to new and synergistic pharmacological approaches independent of control of smooth muscle cell proliferation, which appears to be an early process and, consequently, difficult to limit.

What Causes Smooth Muscle Cell Proliferation

Smooth muscle cell proliferation in response to injury of the blood vessel wall is a complex and intricate process which has not yet been satisfactorily clarified. Studies employing various animal models to simulate the postangioplasty environment have revealed that balloon denudation in arteries will initiate a particular biological cascade if either of two pre-requisite conditions are present: (1) extensive endothelial denudation or (2) significant smooth muscle cell injury.

The pioneering work of Reidy et al. demonstrated that significant intimal hyperplasia occurs following balloon injury in rat carotid arteries, which results in the loss of up to 25% of the vessel wall DNA [55, 56]. This loss reflects widespread medial smooth muscle cell injury since endothelial cell loss alone could not account for such a major change in DNA content. Subsequently, more sophisticated techniques of inducing vessel wall injury enabled discrete localization to the endothelium, sparing the subendothelial and medial layers. Intimal overgrowth was only observed in vessel regions which were not completely re-endothelialized by 7 days [74]. These studies, interestingly, suggested that the proliferation and migration of smooth smooth muscle cells are under separate control since some areas of rapid endothelial regrowth contained increased numbers of medial smooth muscle cells but without a corresponding increase in intimal thickness. This theory is supported by a series of autoradiographic experiments which illustrated that only 50% of intimal smorth muscle cells are capable of proliferation [75, 76].

Growth Factors in Restenosis

Many structurally distinct substances have been implicated as mitogens or cytokines or chemotactic agents in the biological cascade which ultimately leads to smooth muscle cell proliferation. Platelet-derived growth factor (PDGF), the most intensively studied factor, is a dimer compound composed to two homologous polypeptide chains (A and B) linked by a disulphide bond [77]. Although PDGF was originally isolated from platelets, further study has confirmed that it is also released by several other cells, including vascular endothelium, macrophages, and even activated smooth muscle cells, which may explain why smooth muscle cells continue to proliferate long after the initial platelet–vessel wall interaction [78–81].

The binding of PDGF to its receptor initiates a complex cascade of signal transduction within the cytoplasm, and ultimately within the nucleus of the smooth muscle cell, resulting in cell division and protein synthesis. Although these pathways have not been fully elucidated, the PDGF-receptor mediated phosphorylation of tyrosine kinase, which then activates phospholipase C, which subsequently generates two important second messengers (diacylglycerol and inositol triphosphate) [82, 83], is certainly an important step. The PDGF receptor and both chains of PDGF have been sequenced, and it is now possible to clone PDGF using recombinant technology. Monoclonal antibodies against both chains of PDGF and its receptor have also been produced. The gene that codes for the B chain mRNA of PDGF is c-*sis*, which is the cellular counterpart to the v-*sis* gene of the simian sarcoma virus. The demonstration of an active human oncogene in atherosclerotic plaques has unveiled an intriguing connection between atherosclerosis and oncogenesis [84]. Cultured mouse fibroblast NIH 3T3 cells have been transformed with transfected DNA from these plaques [85], leading to the development of slow growing tumours in "nude" mice.

Other important growth factors reputed to play a role in the restenosis process include interleukin-1 (IL-1), fibroblast growth factor (FGF), colony stimulating factor (CSF), epidermal growth factor (EGF), transforming growth factor-β, insulin-like growth factor (somatomedins), endothelin and serotonin. These compounds may have overlapping and/or multiple functions; their possible interactions are unknown and consequently their relative influence is completely speculative. Such an extent of uncertainty illustrates our limited understanding of the entire process.

Pathological Time Course of Restenosis According to Current Knowledge

It is now believed that following ballon injury, denudation of endothelial cells is rapidly followed by platelet adhesion and aggregation, with the release of a plethora of substances, including the previously mentioned growth factors, most notably PDGF and FGF [86]. These two mitogens may, respectively, prime smooth muscle and endothelial cells for the actions of other factors, culminating in DNA synthesis [87]. Endothelial cells and medial smooth muscle cells are, in turn, rendered receptive to these various growth factors by the cleavage of heparin proteoglycan from their surfaces by an endoglycosidase released by activated platelets [70]. The released heparin is thought to be potently chemotactic for growth factors and further increase their local concentration in a powerful synergistic cascade, resulting in transformation of smooth muscle cells to the synthetic phenotype [86, 88].

Smooth muscle cells begin to proliferate first in the media [70], but by day 4 begin to migrate into the damaged area [55, 56, 89] and start to produce chondroitin sulphate and dermatan sulphate proteoglycans when they reach the myointimal space [90]. Simultaneously, endothelial cells migrate from the lateral edges of the denuded intima [56, 89], promoted by FGF [91] and facilitated by fibronectin and hyaluronic acid present in the extracellular matrix [90]. The damaged area may, depending on its size, be resurfaced by a new layer of endothelial cells by day 7 [74, 75]. Reidy has suggested that if the denuded area is less than 1 cm long, then intimal hyperplasia does not ensue [74, 92]. It is likely, therefore, that there is a critical area of intimal disruption, and perhaps time-window, for endothelial cells to provide a complete covering before maximal smooth muscle cell proliferation begins, with consequent possibilities for inhibition or retardation of this process.

As the new intact blood vessel surface is completed, endothelial cells, having stopped proliferating, begin to synthesize heparin proteoglycan [93], which is retained by the intact endothelial layer and accumulates rapidly within the myointimal space. Smooth muscle cells bind heparin, which inhibits their proliferation by rendering them unresponsive to growth factors [88], but potentiates further extracellular matrix production by activating TGF-β [94]. Two weeks following injury, some synthetic smooth muscle cells begin to adopt a contractile appearance [54, 89], and this pattern progresses at a rate depending on a number of factors, particularly the extent of injury, and is in parallel with the gradual replacement of proteoglycan in the extracellular matrix by collagen [72] during the succeeding months. Throughout this period, the characteristic histological appearance of intimal hyperplasia is observed, i.e., proliferating smooth muscle cells in varying concentrations against a background of a loose matrix largely composed of proteoglycan [54].

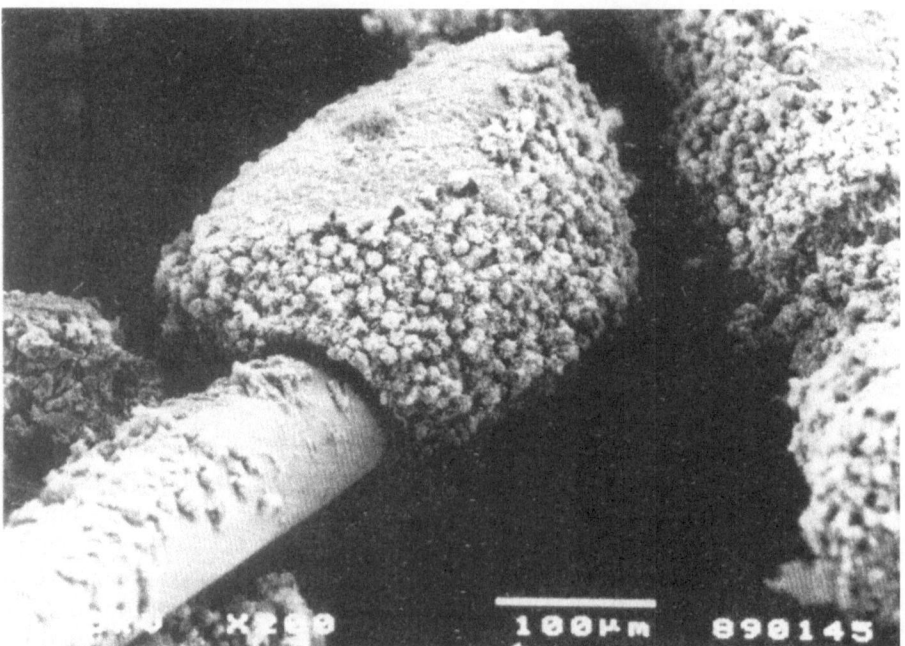

Fig. 2. Scanning electron micrograph of a stented human saphenous vein bypass graft retrieved between 3–7 days after implantation. There is obvious extensive deposition of platelets, leukocytes and fibrin on the featured stent filament

By 6 months, basal conditions of the pre-injury vessel wall are restored, with intact endothelial layer and predominance of contractile smooth muscle cells in a mainly collagenous matrix [89, 95]. In some cases, in which there was extensive injury with chronic persistent endothelial denudation, proliferative cell types may predominate beyond this time and intimal hyperplasia continues [56, 96].

Pathology of Restenosis: Is It the Same for Stents?

We have retrieved and examined stented venous bypass grafts from several patients and, in addition, a number of observational animal studies exploring the pathology of restenosis in stents have been carried out by our group. Although the extent of intimal hyperplasia is similar to postangioplasty examination, several histological features appear to be unique to the stenting situation.

Extensive deposition of platelets, fibrin and leucocytes was observed along the stent wires in human saphenous vein bypass grafts and porcine

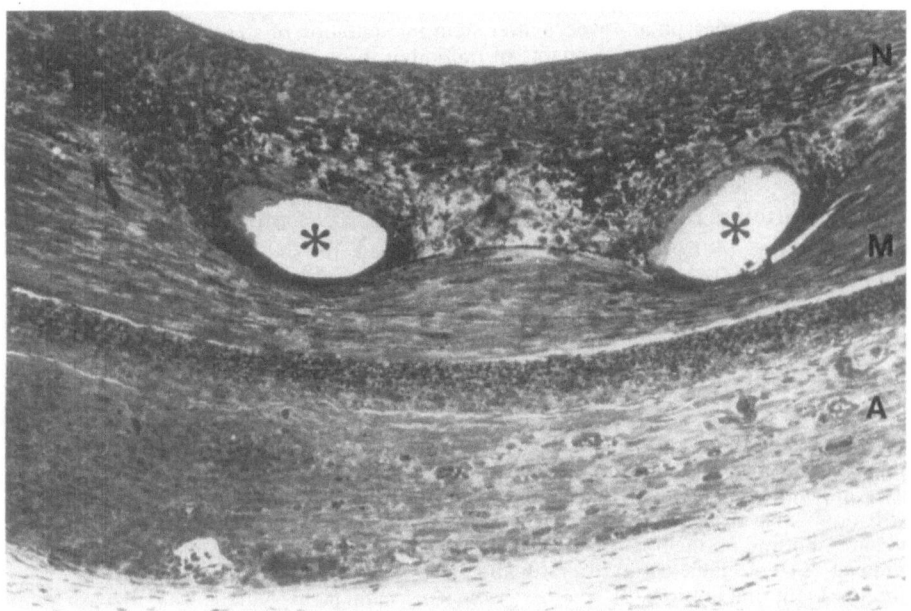

Fig. 3. Light micrograph of stented porcine coronary artery at 7 days. The *clear circular areas* marked (*) are the sites of the stent wires of 70μ in diameter which have been removed. There is a disorganized layer of neointima (N) on the luminal aspect of these clear areas which is composed of smooth muscle cells, trapped red blood cells and fibrin. Above this is an organized neointima of smooth muscle cells covered by endothelium. The internal elastic lamina is interrupted as indicated by the *arrow*. M, media; A, adventitia

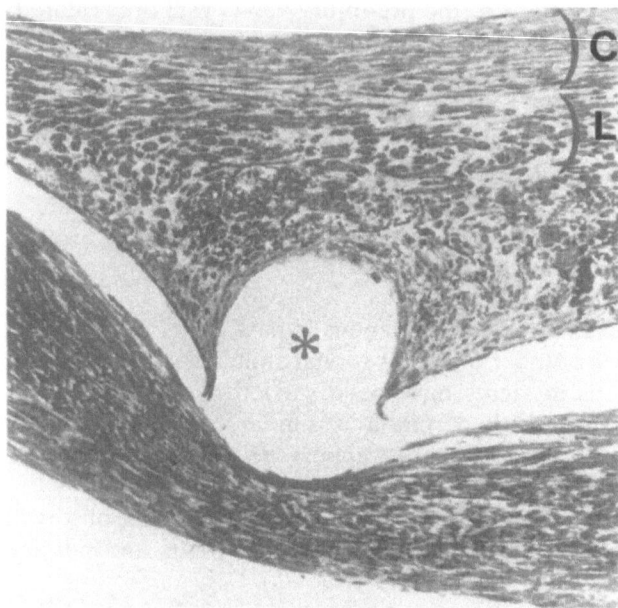

Fig. 4. Light micrograph at 4 weeks after stent implantation of a cross section of porcine coronary artery showing the remnants of the initial thrombus, which now contains some erythrocytes, leukocytes and lipid laden foam cells interspersed throughout a disorganized fibrocellular layer. On the luminal side, two distinct layers of smooth muscle cells are obvious, a superficial layer with circular orientation (*C*) and a deeper, longitudinally orientated layer (*L*). *, space created following removal of a stent wire 70 μ in diameter

coronary arteries retrieved 3–7 days following stent implantation (Fig. 2). In the pigs, the stent wires become embedded in the vessel wall and are covered with a neointima within 7 days. This neointima consists of organizing thrombus directly adherent to the wire and several layers of smooth muscle cells along the luminal surface (Fig. 3). Scanning electron microscopy confirms complete endothelialization.

⟶

Fig. 5. Light micrograph of a cross section of stented porcine coronary artery 3 months after implantation. Compared with Fig 4, a much more extensive neointima is evident with only small areas of leukocyte aggregation and cellular debris, as indicated by the *arrows*, abutting on the sites of the removed stent filaments *, space remaining following removal of stent filaments of 70 μ in diameter

Fig. 6. Light micrograph of a cross section of human saphenous vein bypass graft removed 10 months after stent implantation. The old atherosclerotic plaque (*P*) is separated from the prominent neointimal layer (*N*) by aggregates of abundant foam cells. *, space remaining following removal of stent filament of 70 μ in diameter

Fig. 7a,b. Transmission electron micrograph of another stented saphenous vein bypass graft removed 6 months following implantation. Extracellular lipid deposits and cholesterol clefts (*arrow*) are evident alongside the foam cells. Higher magnification (**b**) of a segment from **a** showing abundant foam cells. *, space remaining following removal of stent filament of 70 μ in diameter. *P*, plaque; *N*, neointima

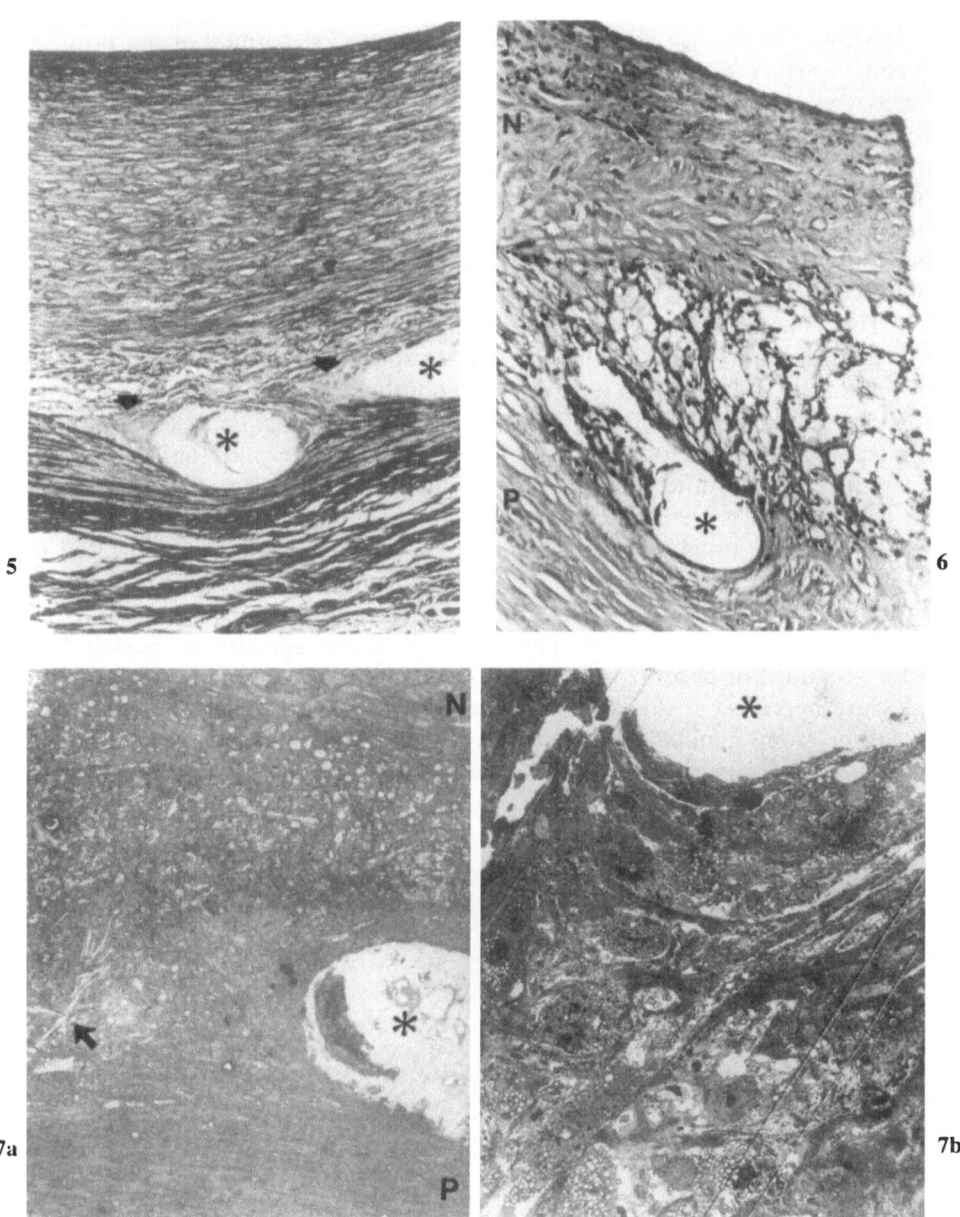

At 4 weeks in porcine coronary arteries, few traces remain of the initial platelet–fibrin thrombus, which by then has been replaced by erythrocytes, leucocytes and lipid-laden foam cells which are interspersed throughout a disorganized fibrocellular layer (Fig. 4). At the luminal side, two distinct layers of smooth muscle cells are present, one in a circular orientation immediately below the endothelium and a deeper layer in a longitudinal orientation.

After 3 months, a more extensive neointima has formed in the porcine coronary artery with only a small area adjacent to the stent wire containing leucocytes and cellular debris (the so-called Bermuda Triangle, Fig. 5). In human saphenous vein grafts removed 3–10 months after the stenting procedure, a comparable amount of neointima has developed as in the pigs, but it borders on the old atherosclerotic plaque (Fig. 6). At the junction between old plaque and neointima, abundant foam cells and extracellular lipid deposits are found, in addition to extensive extracellular matrix production (Fig. 7A,B).

The causes and possible relationships between these early and later histological features are unknown. We are speculating that two factors may be important. Firstly, the regenerated endothelium that covers the stented segment may be dysfunctional and thus permit abnormal and excessive lipid infiltration and macrophage penetration across the endothelial barrier. Scanning electron microscopy (EM) of the endothelial lining has indicated an irregular, raised endothelial surface in lieu of the normal smooth covering (Fig. 8), although no permeability to Evan's Blue was demonstrated in stented porcine arteries after 4 months. Secondly, important chemotactic substances may be released by the cellular debris trapped in the tissue adjacent to the stent wires. This area of debris appears to persist late after stenting for several reasons, including continued damage from direct pressure necrosis, or due to its deeper location in the vessel wall, and thus isolation from laminar flow patterns which predominate on the luminal aspect of the stent wires. A striking similarity exists between the biology of

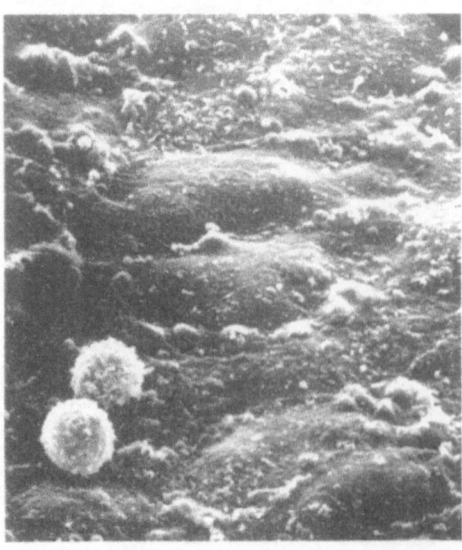

Fig. 8. Scanning electron micrograph of the endothelial surface of the stented bypass graft featured in Fig. 7, revealing it as smooth, raised and irregular. Two leukocytes are adherent to the endothelium

stented vessels at 3 months and chronic atherosclerotic lesions, namely proliferation of smooth muscle cells, large amounts of connective tissue matrix including collagen, elastin and proteoglycans, lipid accumulation in the form of foam cells (smooth muscle cells and macrophages), and extracellular deposits. The natural history of these post stent lesions has yet to be determined.

Unique Features of the Stent Applied to Restenosis

Several possible theories have been proposed to support a role for the endoluminal stent in limiting intimal hyperplasia [33, 97, 98]. There is, however, minimal experimental evidence to justify this position and avail-

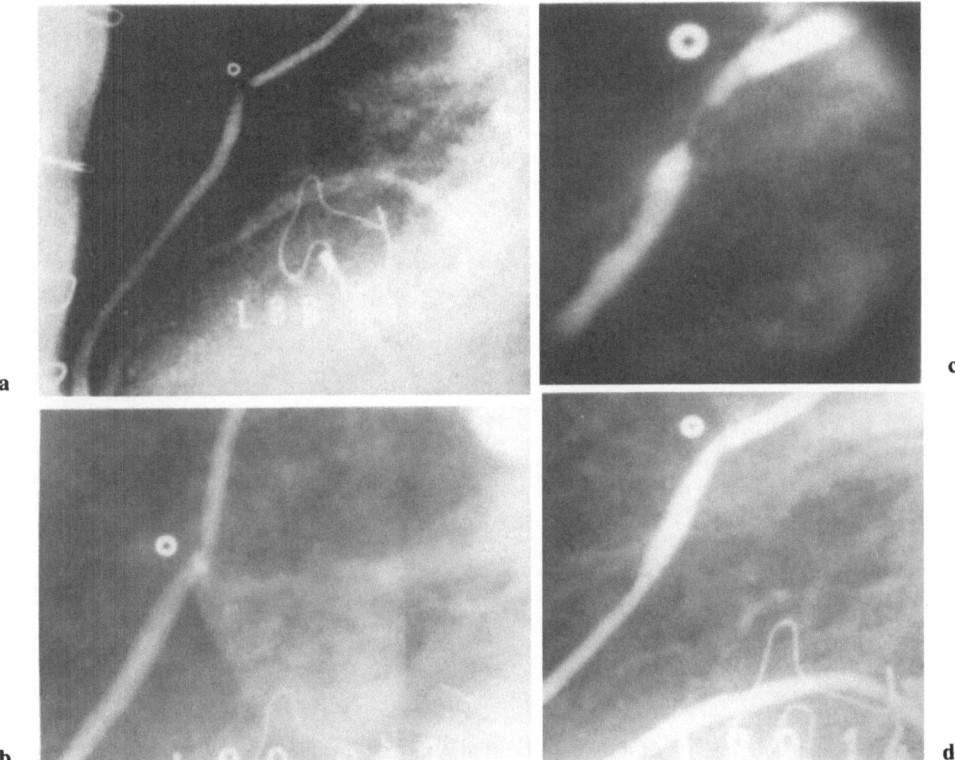

Fig. 9a–d. Coronary angiogram from a 67-year-old patient who underwent stent implantation for a severe narrowing in the shaft of a 10-year-old saphenous vein bypass graft. Three months later he was treated, by atherectomy, for restenosis within the stent. **a** Before stent; **b** immediately following stenting; **c** restenosis at 3 months after stenting; **d** after athesectomy

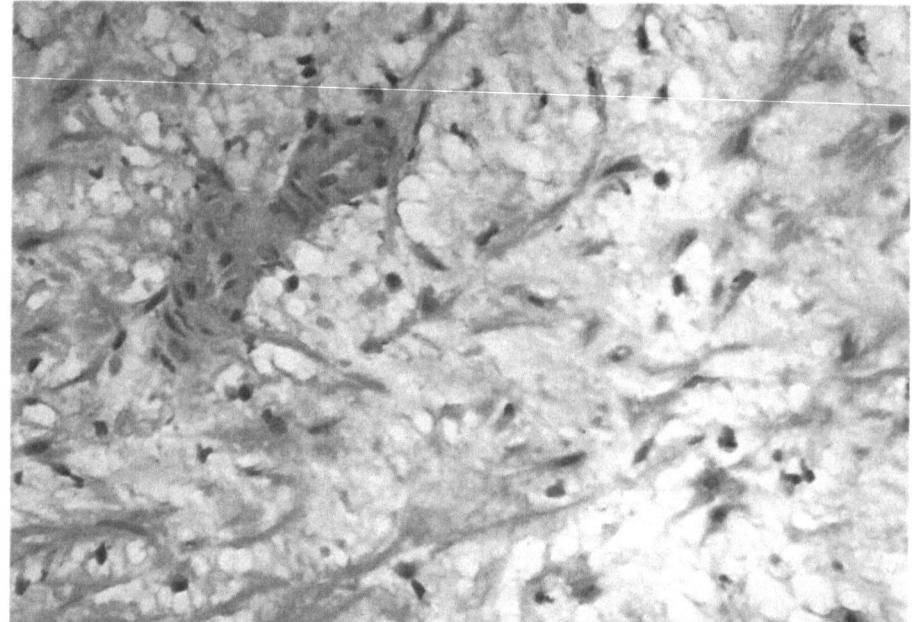

10

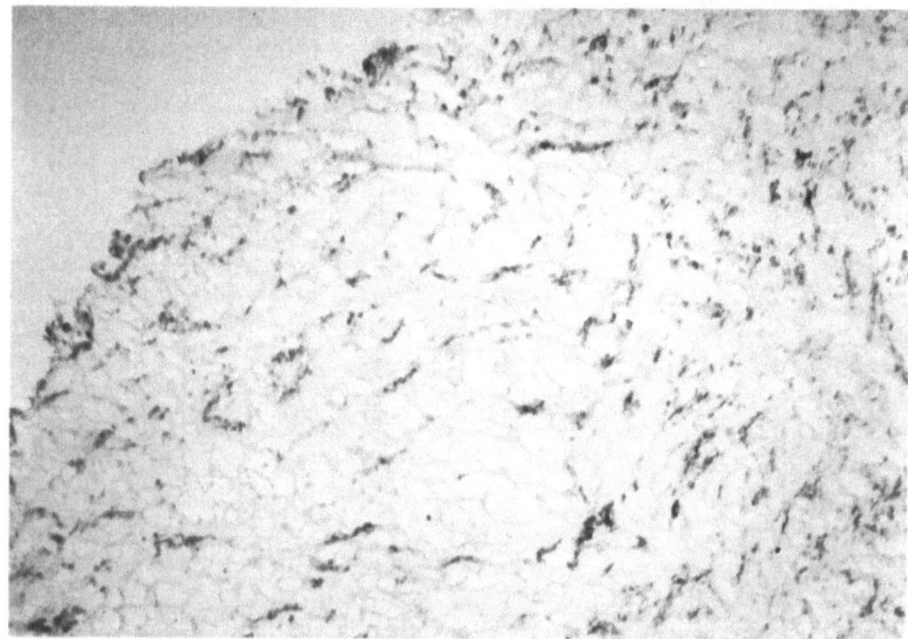

11

Fig. 10. Light micrograph of a tissue specimen removed by atherectomy from the stenosis within the stent featured in Fig. 9 demonstrating abundant smooth muscle cells in a loose extracellular matrix. Two capillaries are also present within the segment. (Hematoxylin and eosin stain)

Fig. 11. An antibody specific for smooth muscle α actin has been coupled with a peroxidase reaction, identifying smooth muscle cells by the dark brown staining seen in this light micrograph of further tissue obtained by atherectomy from the same stent stenosis

able animal and clinical studies demonstrate that significant hyperplasia occurs within the stented segment [99–102]. The extent and characteristics of this hyperplasia are illustrated by the case of a 67-year-old man who had recurrence of angina 3 months following stenting of a bypass graft. Angiography revealed a severe narrowing within the stent which was treated by combined balloon angioplasty and atherectomy (Fig. 9a–d). The tissue specimens removed by the atherectomy device are shown in Fig. 10. Microscopic evaluation showed abundant extracellular collagenous matrix and areas of marked cellularity which stained positively for the two smooth muscle cell cytoskeleton proteins, alpha actin and vimentin (Fig. 11).

Although hyperplasia is a consequence of stenting, the functional significance of this overgrowth may be diminished by the intrinsic dilating property of the self-expanding stent which results in excellent intial improvement in luminal diameter–50% superior to angioplasty alone which, in many patients, more than compensates for the late proliferation [99–101]. Similar immediate improvements in luminal profile have been observed during preliminary experience with the Wiktor stent, a tantalum balloon expandable coil stent [102]. The ideal ratio of stent size to vessel size which will result in optimal dilation with minimal compensatory hyperplasia remains unknown, although recent data from Strauss et al. identify oversizing by over 0.7 mm to be significantly associated with luminal renarrowing after stent implantation [100]. In addition, this elegant paper pointed out that the use of multiple stents per lesion is to be avoided for the same reason [100]. The relationship between overdilatation and hyperplasia and its consequent importance with regard to final outcome has been further characterized by Schwartz et al. by implanting stainless steel mesh stents and tantalum coils, in a porcine model, with markedly oversized PTCA balloons, inflated to pressures of up to 14 atmospheres [103].

There are three unique aspects of stenting which further confound our understanding of the processes occurring in the vessel wall following injury. Firstly, in contrast to the brief, transient injury induced by balloon angioplasty, nonbiodegradable stents are permanent foreign bodies, with potentially important interactions due to the type of metal, electrostatic charges, and possibly physical irritation from individual filaments. Whether the continued presence of a foreign body in the vascular wall will continue to stimulate fibrointimal hyperplasia beyond the 6 months usually associated with balloon injury is also unknown. In addition, concern has been expressed as to whether an allergic response could be triggered by individual stent components in hypersensitive patients. There have been reports of transient inflammatory infiltrates in the adventitia following stent implantation [14, 15], and although up to now there was no evidence to fortify a hypothesis for an additional contribution by a foreign body reaction, our group has recently opened this aspect of the wound, by identifying and documenting the presence of multinucleated giant cells in the vicinity of stent wires in a saphenous vein graft retrieved during repeat coronary

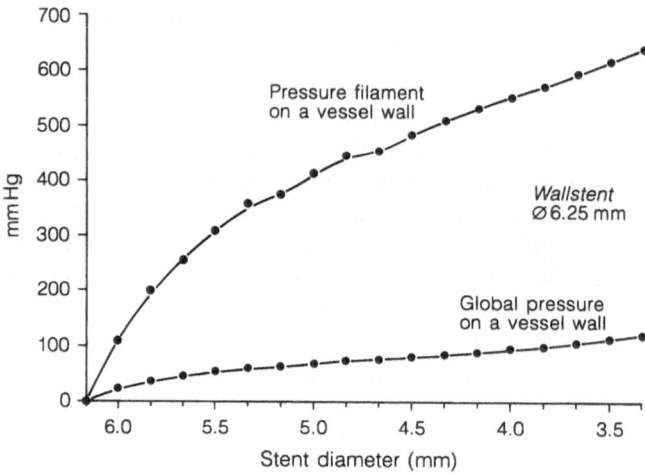

Fig. 12. Radial pressures exerted by individual stent filaments and the global pressure exerted by the entire device (a self-expandable Wallstent – unconstrained diameter 6.25 mm) on the vessel wall at varying degrees of expansion (see text for explanation)

artery bypass operation 85 days after stent implantation (unpublished observations). In vitro attempts by our group to identify endothelial membrane lipid peroxidation by free radicals formed in the presence of stent metallic elements (Fe, Cu) have been unsuccessful, although the theoretical possibility exists.

Secondly, the chronic effects of continuous barotrauma induced by the expanded stent may have important ramifications. Since it has properties analogous to any spring, the Wallstent will attempt to assume its equilibrium configuration (defined as the unconstrained diameter where net radial force is zero), if it is stretched or constricted. We have studied the force–length relationship of the Wallstent at varying degrees of stretch, which correspondingly alter the diameter of stent (Fig. 12). From these measurements, it is possible to calculate the radial pressures exerted by the stent, both globally and locally at the site of the individual filaments if the stent is maintained at a diameter which is less than the unconstrained diameter. Considerable pressures are generated by the stent (as in any spring-loaded device) to return it to its unconstrained size. For example, an unconstrained stent 6.25 mm in diameter generates a radial pressure globally of 50 mmHg and about 300 mmHg locally at the stent filament if it is maintained at 5.5 mm. This increases to 90 mm globally and 500 mm locally at 4.5 mm diameter. These pressures are likely to be additive with mean arterial pressure and could have an important impact in situations in which over-sized Wallstents are implanted. In fact, we have occasionally noted localized areas of vessel wall necrosis adjacent to stent wires, which, we believe, are probably the result of a pressure phenomenon.

Thirdly, parallels have been drawn between the effects of splinting the artery externally (termed "casting") and internally (i.e. stenting). Thrubiker et al. have shown that externally casting segments of rabbit aorta limits pulsatile flow and atheroma development, despite a high cholesterol diet [104]. Based on this observation, some authors have speculated that non-flexible internal stents may also reduce wall stress and consequently diminish hyperplasia formation [33]. This analogy is not altogether valid. Although some of the pulsatile stretch may be borne by the external cast or the internal stent, and thus favourably affect wall stress, this is achieved by separate means. In the casting model, there should be a reduction in intramural wall stress, since the vessel is casted at a radius smaller than the maximal systolic expansion. In contrast, internal stenting results in dilatation of the artery and an increase in wall stress. This important stimulus to intimal hyperplasia appears to overcome the inhibitory effects of reduction in phasic vessel wall expansion. Booth and colleagues have modified the external casting model with interesting results [105]. Using an external, nonoccluding, silastic collar, which does not affect end systolic dimensions of the (rabbit carotid) artery, focal hyperplastic lesions were observed to rapidly develop, supporting the concept that external casting must decrease the vessel radius in order to achieve inhibition of intimal hyperplasia.

An Alternative Paradigm for Restenosis

A completely different pathological scheme of things has very recently been proposed by Schwartz et al. [106] based on their observations in a porcine coronary restenosis model [107]. In this model, mural thrombus is identified as having a major role in the determination of neointimal mass. An endothelial lining forms a thin cover over the luminal aspect of the thrombus within 3 days of injury, and smooth muscle cells are first identified, at 7 days, immediately under this new endothelium, growing subsequently downward toward the media, with gradual resorption of thrombus and enlargement of the maturing neointima. This "inside-out" mechanism for restenosis, as it has been termed by its proponents, has many compelling features, particularly the central role of mural thrombus. Its further exploration and characterization, with special emphasis on its applicability to the human situation, is likely to be vitally important in the extension of our understanding of the complex pathophysiological mechanisms underlying the process of response of the vessel wall to iatrogenic injury, the only abiding feature of which – not to put too fine a point on it – is our continued failure to provide satisfactory answers to the multitudinous perplexing questions.

Interventional Cardiology in the 1900s: The Quest for an Ideal Revascularization Technique and the "Niche" Concept

Percutaneous transluminal coronary revascularization procedures continue to increase in popularity and are now competing, not only with CABG, but with each other, for the blue riband of the ideal treatment for obstructive coronary artery disease. Such competition has, of course, positive and negative aspects. On the credit side, any potential for improvement in the success rates of the various modalities will be brought about more rapidly, and similarly, the major drawbacks can be expected to reveal themselves simultaneously. Unfortunately, the negative aspect is that it will become clear, in retrospect, that many patients have been inappropriately assigned to a particular treatment modality with consequent avoidable mortality, in addition to the already mitotic problem of restenosis, but, such is the price of advancement. At the present time, the percutaneous treatment options may be divided into two groups according to the their basic modes of action, i.e. devices which primarily dilate coronary narrowings (balloon angioplasty – with or without "heat" – and endoluminal stenting) and those which physically debulk coronary tissue by extraction, liquefaction or vaporization (laser, directional and rotational atherectomy, and spark erosion). Despite the fact that all of these modalities have been in clinical use for more than 4 years, it is difficult to make comparisons between them with regard to outcome, since randomized trials have only been recently commenced. There are, however, several fundamental differences which are of undoubted, if somewhat undetermined, importance and therefore merit further discussion.

The ideal coronary intervention should selectively improve luminal dimensions with minimal alteration of the normal vessel wall components and architecture. None of the currently available techniques completely satisfy these requirements. Balloon angioplasty, atherectomy (rotational and directional), and laser devices all cause extensive traumatic changes within the plaque, and, usually, major alterations to the vessel wall architecture as well. Balloon angioplasty, the earliest intervention, has been shown to create tears and dissections within and at the edges of atherosclerotic plaques and frequently disrupts the internal elastic membrane and medial layers [68, 108–112]. Theoretically, this may be advantageous since the liberation of lipid and debris from the atheromatous lesions, a sort of debridement, may favourably affect the long-term biological growth and behaviour (if distal embolization of this material does not cause immediate clinical consequences) [113–115]. The manner in which the healing process ensues, in a damaged vessel with frayed, ragged membrane edges and separated muscular layers, and the inherent problems of restoring the normal three-layered architecture of the arterial wall in an orderly fashion after such injury, however, presents a more important mystery for consideration. Furthermore, the extent of arterial disruption, as a consequence of balloon dilatation during angioplasty, appears to be much less than that imparted by the actual removal of coronary tissue by debulking devices. Directional atherectomy, in particular, has been shown to be extremely effective in removing atheroma, and although specimens retrieved may include adventitia in more than 30% of cases [116, 117], there is no strong evidence to date that subsequent restenosis is related to the depth of penetration of the vessel wall [117]. Stenting, on the contrary, seems to be the least disruptive to the underlying architecture, although the primary atheromatous lesion persists in the stented vessel with, as yet, unknown long-term consequences. Cracks and tears induced by balloon angioplasty can be "tacked back" by stenting, theoretically diminishing the stimulus for fibrosis, in a similar manner to the minimization of epidermal fibrotic scar formation during the healing phase, by careful apposition of wound edges at primary closure.

Glagov and colleagues observed that the diseased coronary artery, in order to maintain an adequate lumen, can adapt to progressive plaque expansion by the concomitant enlarging of the vessel [118]. This compensatory mechanism maintains the luminal area until the plaque lesion occupies approximately 40% of the area inside the internal elastic lamina, beyond which point progressive luminal narrowing tends to occur. In other words, significant atherosclerosis can coexist with normal or even enlarged luminal area until the limits of this adaptive process are exceeded.

Striking similarities exist between the chronic process of atherosclerosis and the situation in the stented vessel wall. The stent is initially embedded in the intima which acutely results in enlargement of the lumen and later in localized medial thinning at the site of the stent wires, which is a commonly observed pathologic feature of atherosclerosis. Stenting may be regarded as the invasive cardiologist's attempt to restore the aforementioned "Glagovian" balance between plaque and luminal area, but now in vessels which contain plaques exceeding 40% of the internal elastic lamina (Fig. 12). Stents effectively alter the relationship between plaque size and lumen area, resulting in a shift in the curve. Progressive vessel dilatation by the stent can maintain adequate luminal area unless excessive fibrointimal hyperplasia upsets the new balance.

Expansion Ratio

Expansion ratio is an important concept that relates the final effect of the device on the arterial diameter to the size of the catheter required to deliver this effect [33] (Table 2). A favourable ratio is best exemplified by a small catheter delivery system which can traverse severely narrowed segments and yet optimally dilate or ablate the stenosis. The maximum effect of the device may be partially lost due to the elastic recoil of the vessel. The current interventional devices may have differential effects in these two areas: the

Table 2. Expansion ratios with the interventional devices

Intervention	Procedures	Device profile (mm)	Pre-procedure vessel diameter (mm)	Maximum achievable diameter (mm)	Post-procedure diameter (mm)	Theoretical expansion ratio	Effective expansion ratio
Balloon angioplasty	443	0.7–1.3	1.1 ± 0.3	2.9 ± 0.4 (2.0–3.5)	1.8 ± 0.4	2.2–4.1	1.4–2.6
Stent							
Self-expandable	357	1.6	1.3 ± 0.7	4.0 ± 0.7 (2.5–6.0)	2.6 ± 0.6	2.5 (1.6–3.8)	1.6
Balloon expandable	95	1.4–1.6	1.1 ± 0.3	3.3 ± 0.3 (3.0–4.0)	2.4 ± 0.3	2.1–2.4	1.5–1.7
Atherectomy							
Directional	122	2.1–2.5	1.1 ± 0.4	3.3 ± 0.5[a] / 2.0 ± 0.2[b]	2.5 ± 0.6	1.3–1.6	1.0–1.2
Rotational	52	1.5–2.0	0.9 ± 0.3	1.9 ± 0.3 (1.5–2.0)	1.7 ± 0.4	1.0	0.9–1.1
Excimer laser	55	1.4	0.5 ± 0.4	1.4	1.7 ± 0.5	1.0	1.2

This table compares the device profile and immediate angiographic results of several interventions. The profile of the device is based on data on 2.0–3.5 mm diameter balloon catheters [133], the Wallstent (Medinvent) self-expandable stent, Wiktor (Medtronic) balloon expandable stent, Simpson Coronary Atherocath (DVI) directional atherectomy, Rotablator (Heart Technology) rotational atherectomy and the Model Max-10 excimer laser (Technolas, Munich). The relationship between the profile of the device and the maximum achievable diameter of the device is the theoretical expansion ratio. The maximum achievable diameter of the vessel is calculated according to the size of the device while it is operational in the coronary vessel. In the case of balloon angioplasty, balloon expandable stent, and directional atherectomy, this corresponds to the diameter of the device while the balloon is inflated and to the unconstrained diameter of the self-expandable stent. The rotational atherectomy and the excimer laser do not alter their diameter during the procedure. The post-procedure diameter was measured immediately following the procedure. The effective expansion ratio represents the ratio between the post-procedure result and the profile of the device and thus indicates not only the initial effect of the device but also the effect of elastic recoil which is primarily responsible for the deterioration in the diameter between the maximum achievable diameter and the post-procedure diameter. The diameter values listed are the mean and standard deviation of the different sized devices from each interventional study with the ranges included in the brackets. The pre-procedure data, which may also effect the post-procedural result, were similar for all interventions (0.9–1.3 mm) except the excimer laser, which may explain a somewhat lower post recoil diameter and effective expansion ratio. The quantitative angiographic data for all devices were collected at the Thoraxcenter with the exception of the rotational atherectomy (Kirk Peterson, personal communication) and the excimer laser [134].

NA, not available. [a] With balloon inflated. [b] With balloon deflated.

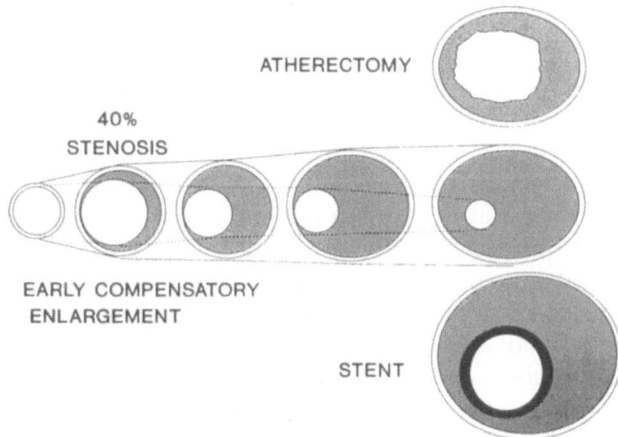

Fig. 13. Natural progression of coronary artery disease as suggested by Glagov, with early compensatory enlargement and late luminal narrowing of progressive atherosclerosis. The contrasting effects of stenting and atherectomy in the restoration of the vessel lumen are illustrated. Stenting (bottom) reproduces the early compensatory enlargement of the vessel, similar to Glagov's model, while maintaining the basic architecture of the vessel wall. Alternatively atherectomy (*top*), although restoring similar luminal dimensions, disrupts the underlying architecture of the wall by extracting vascular tissue (modified from [118])

acute result, when the device is initially used, and then the partial loss of the initial gain after the device has been removed. We have attempted to separate these two effects by subdividing the expansion ratio into the theoretical expansion ratio, which is a measure of the effect while the device is operational, and the functional expansion ratio, which takes into account the elastic recoil phenomenon. For example, a balloon angioplasty catheter 4 mm in diameter should achieve a vessel diameter of 4 mm at the time of balloon inflation but this is reduced immediately after deflation, primarily due to the elastic recoil of the vessel. Balloon angioplasty and stenting give extremely favourable theoretical and effective expansion ratios since they may be delivered on low profile catheters. The wide range for the theoretical and effective expansion ratios seen with balloon angioplasty is explained by the varying sized balloons (2.0–3.5 mm) used in the study from which this data was obtained. The atherectomy devices are more limited by the profile of the device which can be introduced into the coronary artery. The dimensions of the rotational atherectomy device and the excimer laser do not change while in operation and therefore both exhibit lower theoretical expansion ratios. However, by physically removing or vaporizing tissue, the potential elastic recoil effect is diminished by atherectomy and excimer laser devices.

The Niche Concept

At this moment in time there is no "ideal" intracoronary treatment modality
and such a concept can be dispelled as a myth. All available modalities are
attended by similar general early success and complication "rates" [119]
and cannot improve on those now offered by PTCA. Restenosis is still
the Achilles heel of this approach to the treatment of coronary disease.
The recently highlighted value of laser therapy at plaque erosion in particular circumstances (such as chronic occlusions, calcified, long, irregular or
ostial coronary lesions [120]) and of directional atherectomy in concentric
"restenotic" lesions and "complex lesions appearing to contain thrombus"
(especially in saphenous vein grafts) [121] has unveiled perhaps a new
concept in interventional cardiology – a "niche" for each of the treatment modalities [119]. This would imply only minimal overlap between
recommendations of appropriateness for a particular modality and therefore rationalization of approach and consequent increase in the number of
patients previously labelled as having "unsuitable anatomy" (currently
about 50%), in whom a non-surgical intervention might offer a reasonable
alternative to medical therapy or coronary artery bypass grafting.

The place of the stent in this scheme remains to be defined. Widespread
acceptance will only be achieved when the safety, efficacy and cost efficiency
is superior to balloon angioplasty alone. Although there is obvious and
definite improvement, safety remains a major concern. In the initial 105
patients treated by implantation of a Wallstent, 20% had documented occlusions within the first 14 days, usually resulting in myocardial infarction
and in some cases necessitating emergency bypass surgery. With further
experience this was reduced to 13% in the next 100 patients. Schatz and
colleagues recently reported a 3.6% subacute occlusion rate in contrast
to 16% in their early experience, when warfarin treatment was omitted
[122]. Preliminary European experience with the Wiktor stent yielded a
subacute/acute occlusion rate of 11%, with the majority of these patients
being successfully treated by thrombolysis ±PTCA, without recourse to
emergency CABG [102]. Subacute stent occlusion has properly become the
focus of much recent attention. Some studies have attempted to identify
angiographic predictors of this troublesome occurrence, which is reported
in 5%–17% of patients receiving an intracoronary stent for acute vessel
closure following PTCA, or as elective treatment for coronary stenosis or
restenosis [123–127]. Angiographic identification of thrombus, before or
after stenting, or of the presence of residual intimal dissection, or of a
suboptimal angiographic result after stent implantation have been shown to
be associated with an increased risk of subacute occlusion [123, 124]. Global
anticoagulation tests are unable to predict these events [125], but more
specific monitoring of anticoagulation therapy appears to be superior and
may lead to a reduction in subacute thrombotic occlusion [126], as may
more aggressive or potent anticoagulation [123]. Treatment by thrombolysis

with, or without, additional PTCA, avoiding the need for emergency CABG, is successful and satisfactory in the majority of cases [102, 125].

The cost of necessarily rigid chronic anticoagulation therapeutic regimes in terms of bleeding complications, prolonged hospitalizations to initiate therapy, effects on the quality of life, and the consequent obligatory exclusion of otherwise "suitable" patients deemed or predicted (for whatever reason) to have low compliance, must also be considered.

Long-Term Clinical Outcome After Stenting

At the core laboratory associated with our institution, follow-up data have been prospectively gathered on more than 500 patients treated by stent implantation. Analysis of this data reveals perhaps more difficulties than conclusive observations. It is possible to state that both the Wallstent and Wiktor stent achieve similar improvements in stenosis luminal dimensions [128]. Comparison of long-term outcome of the Wallstent with PTCA in "matched" lesions (where the preprocedural location, reference diameter and minimal luminal diameter are identical, within the range of reproducibility of the quantitative analysis system) concluded that stenting yields a greater luminal diameter at follow-up, despite being attended by a greater loss in luminal diameter during follow-up [129]. Using traditional (>50% diameter stenosis at follow-up) or absolute (deterioration of ≥0.72 mm in minimal luminal diameter during follow-up) categorical criteria for angiographic restenosis reveals a wide discrepancy in the assessment of outcome – restenosis rates of 24% and 35%, respectively, among 179 patients followed up after implantation of Wallstent [100] and of 20% versus 48%, respectively, in a preliminary report of follow-up after Wiktor stent implantation [102]. The most salient feature of these studies is the uncertainty about what constitutes "restenosis", which is, after all, the crucial determinant of outcome. Recently inaugurated prospective, randomized studies will, hopefully, clarify the ultimate role or "niche" of the stent.

Perspectives in Restenosis

Even though the current pathological evidence (as described earlier), despite its limitations and uncertainties, illustrates that restenosis is a continuous process – and this has been borne out by quantitative angiographic studies – most investigators continue to apply categorical criteria to the angiographic "definition" of restenosis. In other words, an attempt is made to identify two separate populations, those with and those without restenosis, by using, for the most part, an arbitrary cut-off point. Rensing et al. have described how luminal renarrowing after balloon angioplasty follows a near

Gaussian (or "normal") distribution [130], which invalidates the creation of two separate populations and demonstrates the fallacy of using "restenosis rate" as the ultimate measure of effectiveness of a treatment modality. Umans et al. [131] and de Jaegere et al. [130] have found matching of coronary lesions to be an extremely useful technique by which to compare the outcome of different interventions. Hermans et al. [132] have described and introduced the concepts of relative gain and loss as a sliding scale to facilitate comparison of outcome following PTCA between vessels of different sizes, by taking the reference diameter of the dilated segment into consideration. As a consequence of these rapidly evolving concepts, we anticipate a major fundamental change in the approach to the angiographic assessment of restenosis in the near future.

A Thought for the Future

The apparently self-contradictory observations arising from the analysis of follow-up data in patients treated with stents, as summarized above, raise another important issue, i.e. what is the final angiographic parameter of interest? Is it the degree of change in luminal diameter *during* follow-up, which is intended to reflect the process of intimal hyperplasia, or is it the corollary – the degree of luminal patency remaining *at* follow-up, since this dictates the efficiency of blood delivery to the myocardium, regardless of the thickness of the wall of the conduit. Perhaps the greatest challenge to interventionalists will not be the mastering of techniques or the assignment of each of the treatment modalities to an appropriate "niche", but rather how to derive a universally acceptable method of describing the outcome of these interventions. The champions of quantitative coronary angiography, coronary flow reserve, absolute coronary blood flow, nuclear imaging, echocardiography (both transthoracic and intravascular), and positron emission tomography continue to joust with each other and among themselves as to the ideal method of assessment of the immediate and long-term results of intervention. The vacuum which exists in this key area represents a considerable stumbling block to progress, which investigators continue to overlook in the compelling quest for the "Holy grail" and the potential immortality beyond. A collaborative effort, using universally accepted and standardized methodology to assess the outcome of prospectively randomized studies is surely the way to surmount the obstacles and realize the dream more rapidly and efficiently than by continued solo pioneering.

Acknowledgements. We express our gratitude to C.J. Slager for the pressure-length measurements on the self-expandable stents, Helene van Loon for histological preparations, and Marie Angèle Morel and Eline Montauban van Swijndregt for the quantitative angiographic analysis.

References

1. Gruentzig AR, Senning A, Siegenthaler WE (1979) Nonoperative dilatation of coronary-artery stenosis: percutaneous transluminal coronary angioplasty. N Engl J Med 301:61–68
2. Carrel A (1912) Results of the permanent intubation of the thoracic aorta. Surg Gyn Obstet 3:245–48
3. Dotter CT (1969) Transluminally placed coil-spring endarterial tube grafts: long-term patency in canine popliteal artery. Invest Radiol 4:329–332
4. Dotter CT, Bushmann RW, McKinney MK, Rösch J (1983) Transluminal expandable nitinol coil stent grafting: preliminary report. Radiology 147:259–260
5. Cragg A, Lund G, Rysavy J, Castaneda-Zuniga W, Amplatz K (1983) Nonsurgical placement of arterial endoprostheses: a new technique using nitinol wire. Radiology 147:261–263
6. Sugita Y, Shimomitsu T, Oku T, Murabayashi S, Kambic HE, Harasaki H, Shirey E, Golding L, Nose Y (1986) Nonsurgical implantation of a vascular ring prosthesis using thermal shape memory Ti/Ni alloy (nitinol wire). Trans Am Soc Artif Intern Organs 32:30–34
7. Sutton CS, Tominaga R, Harasaki H, Emoto H, Oku T, Kambic HE, Skibinski C, Beck G, Hollman J (1990) Vascular stenting in normal and atherosclerotic rabbits. Studies of the intravascular endoprosthesis of titanium-nickel-alloy. Circulation 81:667–683
8. Maass D, Zollikofer CL, Largiader F, Senning A (1984) Radiological follow-up of transluminally inserted vascular endoprostheses: an experimental study using expanding spirals. Radiology 152:659–663
9. Sigwart U, Puel J, Mirkovitch V, Joffre F, Kappenberger L (1987) Intravascular stents to prevent occlusion and restenosis after transluminal angioplasty. N Engl J Med 316:701–706
10. Rousseau H, Puel J, Joffre F, Sigwart U, Duboucher C, Imbert C, Knight C, Kropf L, Wallsten H (1987) Self-expanding endovascular prosthesis: an experimental study. Radiology 164:709–714
11. Puel J, Juilliere Y, Bertrand ME, Rickards AF, Sigwart U, Serruys PW (1988) Early and late assessment in stenosis geometry after coronary arterial stenting. Am J Cardiol 61:546–553
12. Serruys PW, Juilliere Y, Bertrand ME, Puel J, Rickards AF, Sigwart U (1988) Additional improvement of stenosis geometry in human coronary arteries by stenting after balloon dilatation: a quantitative angiographic study. Am J Cardiol 61:71G–76G
13. Palmaz JC, Sibbitt RR, Reuter SR, Tio FO, Rice WJ (1985) Expandable intraluminal graft: a preliminary study. Radiology 156:73–77
14. Palmaz JC, Sibbitt RR, Tio FO, Reuter SR, Peters JE, Garcia F (1986) Expandable intraluminal vascular graft: a feasibility study. Surgery 99:199–205
15. Palmaz JC, Windeler SA, Garcia F, Tio FO, Sibbitt RR, Reuter SR (1986) Atherosclerotic rabbit aortas: expandable intraluminal grafting. Radiology 160:723–726
16. Schatz RA, Palmaz JC, Tio FO, Garcia F, Garcia O, Reuter SR (1987) Balloon-expandable intracoronary stents in the adult dog. Circulation 76:450–457
17. Lawrence DD, Charnsangavej C, Wright KC, Gianturco C, Wallace S (1987) Percutaneous endovascular graft: experimental evaluation. Radiology 163:357–360
18. Duprat G, Wright KC, Charnsangavej C, Wallace S, Gianturco C (1987) Self-expanding metallic stents for small vessels: an experimental evaluation. Radiology 162:469–472
19. Swart de H, Oppen van J, Bär F, Ommen van V, Habets J, Veen van der F, Wellens H (1989) Percutaneous implantation of intracoronary stents in pigs. Eur Heart J 10 [Abstract Suppl]:325

20. Rollins N, Wright KC, Charnsangavej C, Wallace S, Gianturco C (1987) Self-expanding metallic stents: preliminary evaluation in an atherosclerotic model. Radiology 163:739–742
21. Duprat G, Wright KC, Charnsangavej C, Wallace S, Gianturco C (1987) Flexible balloon-expanded stents for small vessels. Radiology 162:276–278
22. Roubin GS, Robinson KA, King III SB, Gianturco C, Block AJ, Brown JE, Siegel RJ, Douglas JS (1987) Early and late results of intracoronary arterial stenting after coronary angioplasty in dogs. Circulation 76:891–897
23. Robinson KA, Roubin GS, Siegel RJ, Black AJ, Apkarian RP, King SB (1988) Intra-arterial stenting in the atherosclerotic rabbit. Circulation 78:646–653
24. van der Giessen WJ, Serruys PW, van Beusekom HM et al. (1991) Coronary stenting with a new, radiopaque, balloon-expandable endoprosthesis in pigs. Circulation 83:1788–1798
25. Barth KH, Virmani R, Strecker EP, Savin MA, Lindish RT, Matsumoto AH, Teitelbaum GP (1990) Flexible tantalum stents implanted in aortas and iliac arteries: effects in normal canines. Radiology 175:97–102
26. Strecker EP, Liermann D, Barth KH, Wolf HRD, Freudenberg N, Berg G, Westphal Tsikuras P, Savin M, Schneider B (1990) Diseases: experimental and clinical results work in progress. Radiology 175:97–102
27. Didier B, Gaspard PH, Delsanti G, Dovis J, Boyer C (1989) Removable vascular stent: tolerance and angiographic patency. An experimental study. Eur Heart J 10 [Abstract Suppl]:325
28. Slepian MJ, Schmidler A (1988) Polymeric endoluminal paving/sealing: a biodegradable alternative to intracoronary stenting. Circulation 78(II):409A
29. Ellis SG, Roubin GS, King SB III, Douglas JS Jr, Shaw RE, Stertzer SH, Myler RK (1988) In-hospital cardiac mortality after acute closure after coronary angioplasty: analysis of risk factors from 8207 procedures. J Am Coll Cardiol 11:211–216
30. Ellis SG, Roubin GS, King SB III, Douglas JS Jr, Weintraub WS, Thomas RG, Cox WR (1988) Angiographic and clinical predictors of acute closure after antive vessel coronary angioplasty. Circulation 77:372–379
31. Simpfendorfer C, Belardi J, Bellamy G, Galan K, Franco I, Hollman J (1987) Frequency, management, and follow-up of patients with acute coronary occlusions after percutaneous transluminal coronary angioplasty. Am J Cardiol 59:267–269
32. Dorros G, Cowley MJ, Simpson J, Bentivoglio LG, Block PC, Bourassa M, Detre K, Gosselin AJ, Gruntzig AR, Kelsey SF, Kent KM, Mock MB, Mullin SM, Myler RK, Passamani ER, Stertzer SH, Williams DO (1983) Percutaneous transluminal coronary angioplasty: report of complications from the National Heart, Lung, and Blood Institute PTCA Registry. Circulation 67:723–730
33. Schatz RA (1989) A view of vascular stent. Circulation 79:445–457
34. Serruys PW, Bertrand M, Kober G et al. (1990) Morphological change of coronary stenosis stented with the Medtronic Wiktor stent. Initial results from the core lab (abstract). Circulation 83 [Abstract Suppl]:A2615
35. Sigwart U, Urban P, Golf S, Kaufmann U et al. (1988) Emergency stenting for acute occlusion after coronary balloon angioplasty. Circulation 88:1121–1127
36. Roubin GS, Douglas JS Jr, Lembo NJ, Black AJ, King SB III (1988) Intracoronary stenting for acute closure following percutaneous transluminal coronary angioplasty (PTCA) (abstract Circulation 78(II):406A
37. Thornton MA, Gruentzig AR, Hollman Y, King BS, Douglas JS (1984) Coumadin and aspirin in the prevention of recurrence after transluminal coronary angioplasty: a randomized study. Circulation 69:721–727
38. Leimgruber PP, Roubin GS, Hollman J et al. (1986) Restenosis after successful coronary angioplasty in patients with single-vessel disease. Circulation 73:710–717
39. Holmes DR Jr, Vliestra RE, Smith HC et al. (1984) Restenosis after percutaneous transluminal coronary angioplasty: a report from the PTCA Registry of the National Heart, Lung and Blood Institute. Am J Cardiol 53:77C–81C

40. Corocos T, David PR, Val PG et al. (1985) Failure of diltiazem to prevent restenosis after percutaneous transluminal coronary angioplasty. Am Heart J 109:926–931
41. Vandormael MG, Deligonul U, Kern MJ et al. (1987) Multilesion coronary angioplasty: clinical and angiographic follow-up. J Am Coll Cardiol 10:246–252
42. Hirshfeld JW, Schwartz SS, Jugo R et al. (1991) Restenosis after coronary angioplasty: a multivariate statistical model to relate lesion and procedural variables to restenosis. J Am Coll Cardiol 18:647–656
43. Reis GJ, Boucher TM, Sipperly ME et al. (1989) Randomised trial of fish oil for prevention of restenosis after coronary angioplasty. Lancet 2:177–181
44. Meyer J, Schmitz HJ, Kiesslich T et al. (1983) Percutaneous transluminal coronary angioplasty in patients with stable and unstable angina pectoris: analysis of early and late results. Am Heart J 106:973–980
45. Fleck E, Dacian S, Dirschinger J, Hall D, Rudolph W (1984) Quantitative changes in stenotic coronary artery lesions during follow-up after PTCA (abstract). Circulation 70 [Suppl II]:11–176
46. Serruys PW, Luijten HE, Beatt KJ et al. (1988) Incidence of restenosis after successful angioplasty: a time related phenomenon: a quantitative angiographic study in 342 consecutive patients at 1, 2, 3 and 4 months. Circulation 77:361–371
47. Nobuyoshi M, Kimura T, Nosaka H et al. (1988) Restenosis after successful percutaneous transluminal coronary angioplasty: serial angiographic follow-up of 299 patients. J Am Coll Cardiol 12:616–623
48. Bourassa MG, Lesperance J, Eastwood C et al. (1991) Clinical, physiologic, anatomic, and procedural factors predictive of restenosis after percutaneous transluminal coronary angioplasty. J Am Coll Cardiol 18:363–376
49. Wijns W, Serruys PW, Reiber JHC (1985) Early detection of restenosis after successful percutaneous transluminal coronary angioplasty by exercise-redistribution thallium scintigraphy. Am J Cardiol 55:357–361
50. Powelson S, Roubin G, Whitworth H, Gruentzig A (1986) Incidence of early restenosis after successful percutaneous transluminal coronary angioplasty. J Am Coll Cardiol 7:63A
50a. Steele PM, Chesebro JH, Stanson AW, Holmes DR et al. (1985) Balloon angioplasty: natural history of the pathophysiological response to injury in a pig model. Circ Res 57:105–112
51. Kohchi K, Takebayashi S, Block PC, Hiroki T, Nobuyoshi M (1987) Arterial changes after percutaneous transluminal angioplasty: results at autopsy. J Am Coll Cardiol 10:592–599
52. Waller BF, Rothbaum DA, Gorfinkel HJ, Ulbright TM, Linnemeier TJ, Berger SM (1984) Morphologic observations after percutaneous transluminal balloon angioplasty of early and late aortocoronary saphenous vein bypass grafts. J Am Coll Cardiol 4:784–792
53. Austin GE, Ratliff NB, Hollman J, Tabei S, Phillips DF (1985) Intimal proliferation of smooth muscle cells as an explanation for recurrent coronary artery stenosis after percutaneous transluminal coronary angioplasty. J Am Coll Cardiol 6:369–375
54. Nobuyoshi M, Kimura T, Ohishi H et al. (1991) Restenosis after percutaneous transluminal coronary angioplasty: pathologic observations in 20 patients. J Am Coll Cardiol 17:433–439
55. Clowes AW, Reidy MA, Clowes MM (1983) Mechanisms of stenosis after arterial injury. Lab Invest 49:208–215
56. Clowes AW, Reidy MA, Clowes MM (1983) Kinetics of cellular proliferation after arterial injury. Smooth muscle cell growth in the absence of endothelium. Lab Invest 49:327–333
57. Campbell GR, Campbell JH (1985) Smooth muscle phenotype changes in arterial wall homeostasis: implications for the pathogenesis of atherosclerosis. Exp Mol Pathol 42:139–162

58. Kocher D, Skalli O, Bloom WS, Gabbiani G (1984) Cytoskeleton of rat aortic smooth muscle cells: normal conditions and experimental intimal thickening. Lab Invest 50:645–652
59. Schwartz SM, Campbell GR, Campbell JH (1986) Replication of smooth muscle cells in vascular disease. Circ Res 58:427–444
60. Rensing BJ, Hermans WRM, Beatt KJ, Laarman GJ, Suryapranata H, van den Brand M, de Feyter PJ, Serruys PW (1990) Quantitative angiographic assessment of elastic recoil after percutaneous transluminal coronary angioplasty. Am J Cardiol 66:1039–1044
61. Hjemdahl-Monsen CE, Ambrose JA, Borrico S et al. (1990) Angiographic patterns of balloon inflation during percutaneous transluminal coronary angioplasty: role of pressure-diameter curves in studying distensibility and elasticity of the stenotic lesion and the mechanism of dilation. J Am Coll Cardiol 16:569–575
62. Rensing BJ, Hermans WR, Strauss BH, Serruys PW (1991) Regional differences in elastic recoil after percutaneous transluminal coronary angioplasty: a quantitative angiographic study. J Am Coll Cardiol 17:34B–38B
63. Isner JM, Rosenfield K, Losordo DW et al. (1991) Combination balloon-ultrasound imaging catheter for percutaneous transluminal angioplasty. Validation of imaging, analysis of recoil, and identification of plaque fracture. Circulation 84:739–754
64. Hermans WR, Rensing BJ, Strauss BH, Serruys PW (1991) Methodological problems related to the quantitative assessment of stretch, elastic recoil, and balloon-artery ratio. Cathet Cardiovasc Diagn (in press)
65. Hanet C, Wijns W, Michel X, Schroeder E (1991) Influence of balloon size and stenosis morphology on immediate and delayed elastic recoil after percutaneous transluminal coronary angioplasty. J Am Coll Cardiol 18:506–511
66. Beatt KJ, Bertrand M, Puel J, Rickards T, Serruys PW, Sigwart U (1989) Additional improvement in vessel lumen in the first 24 hours after stent implantation due to radial dilating force (abstract). J Am Coll Cardiol 13 [Suppl A]:A224
67. Essed CE, van den Brand M, Becker AE (1983) Transluminal coronary angioplasty and early restenosis: fibrocellular occlusion after wall laceration. Br Heart J 49: 393–396
68. Uchida Y, Hasegawa K, Kawamura K. Shibuya I (1989) Angioscopic observation of the coronary luminal changes induced by coronary angioplasty. Am Heart J 117: 769–776
69. Potkin BN, Roberts WC (1988) Effects of coronary angioplasty of atherosclerotic plaques and relation of plaque composition and arterial size to outcome. Am J Cardiol 62:41–50
70. Campbell GR, Campbell JH, Manderson JA, Horrigan S, Rennick RE (1988) Arterial smooth muscle: a multifunctional mesenchymal cell. Arch Pathol Lab Med 112:977–986
71. Strauss BH, van Suylen RJ, Umans VA et al. (1991) Directional atherectomy for treatment of restenosis within coronary stents: clinical, angiographic and histologic results. In: Strauss BH (ed) Coronary stenting as an adjunct to balloon angioplasty. PhD Thesis, Erasmus University, Rotterdam, pp 123–47
72. Diegelmann RF, Rothkopf LC, Cohen IK (1975) Measurement of collagen biosynthesis during wound healing. J Surg Res 19:239–243
73. Keeley FW, Elmoselhi A, Leenen FHH (1991) Effects of antihypertensive drug classes on regression of connective tissue components of hypertension. J Cardiovasc Pharm 17 [Suppl 2]:S64–S69
74. Reidy MA, Fingerle J, Majesky MW (1988) Proliferation of vascular smooth muscle cells in vivo. In: Juckling KE, Frost PHE (eds) Hyperlipidemia and atherosclerosis. Academic, New York, pp 149–164
75. Clowes AW, Schwartz SM (1985) Significance of quiescent smooth muscle migration in the injured rat carotid artery. Circ Res 56:139–145
76. Tada T, Reidy MA (1987) Endothelial regeneration. Arterial injury followed by rapid endothelial repair induces smooth muscle cell proliferation but not intimal thickening. Am J Pathol 129:429–433

77. Ross R, Raines EW, Bowen-Pope DF (1986) The biology of platelet-derived growth factor. Cell 46:155–169
78. Barrett TB, Benditt EP (1987) Sis (platelet-derived growth factor B chain) gene transcript levels are elevated in human atherosclerotic lesions compared to normal artery. Proc Natl Acad Sci USA 84:1099–1103
79. Libby P, Warner SJC, Salomon RN, Ririnyi LK (1988) Production of platelet-derived growth factor-like mitogen by smooth-muscle cells from human atheroma. New Engl J Med 318:1493–1498
80. Wilcox JN, Smith KM, Williams SM, Gordon D (1988) Platelet-derived growth factor mRNA detection in human atherosclerotic plaques by in situ hybridiztion J Clin Invest 82:1134–1143
81. Hart CE, Forstrom JW, Kelly JD, Seifert RA, Smith RA, Ross R, Murray MJ, Bowen-Pope DF (1988) Two classes of PDGF receptor recognize different isoforms of PDGF. Science 240:1529–1531
82. Druker J, Mamon HJ, Roberts TM (1989) Oncogenes, growth factors and signal transduction. New Engl J Med 20:1383–1391
83. Mitchell RH (1989) Post-receptor signalling pathways. Lancet 1:765–769
84. Scott J (1987) Oncogenes in atherosclerosis. Nature 325:574–575
85. Penn A, Garte SJ, Warner L, Nesta D, Mindich B (1986) Transforming gene in human atherosclerotic plaque DNA. Proc Natl Acad Sci USA 83:6844–6848
86. Lobb RR (1988) Clinical applications of heparin-binding growth factors. Eur J Clin Invest 18:321–336
87. Walker LN, Bowen-Pope DF, Ross R, Reidy MA (1986) Production of platelet-derived growth factor-like molecules by cultured arterial smooth muscle cells accompanies proliferation after arterial injury. Proc Natl Acad Sci USA 83: 7311–7315
88. Castellot JJ, Wright TC, Karnovsky MJ (1987) Regulation of vascular smooth muscle cell growth by heparin and heparin sulfates. Semin Thromb Hemost 12: 489–503
89. Campbell JH, Campbell GR (1986) Endothelial cell influences on vascular smooth muscle phenotype. Annu Rev Physiol 48:295–306
90. Bently JP (1967) Rate of chondroitin sulfate formation in wound healing. Ann Surg 165:186–191
91. Folkman J, Klagsbrun M (1987) Angiogenic factors. Science 234:442–447
92. Reidy MA, Schwartz SM (1981) Endothelial regeneration. III. Time course of intimal change after small defined injury to rat endothelium. Lab Invest 44:301–308
93. Bassols A, Massague J (1988) Transforming growth factor beta regulates the expression and structure of extracellular matrix chondroitin/dermatan sulfate proteoglycans. J Biol Chem 263:3039–3045
94. McCaffrey TA, Falcone DJ, Brayton CF, Agarwal LA, Welt FGP, Weksler BB (1989) Transforming growth factor-beta-activity is potentiated by heparin via dissociation of the transforming growth factor beta/alpha-macroglobulin inactive complex. J Cell Biol 109:441–448
95. Manderson JA, Moose PRL, Satstrom JA, Young SB, Campbell GR (1989) Balloon catheter injury to rabbit carotid artery. I. Changes in smooth muscle phenotype. Arteriosclerosis 9:289–296
96. Clowes AW, Clowes MM, Reidy MA (1986) Kinetics of cellular proliferation after arterial injury. III. Endothelial and smooth muscle growth in chronically denuded vessels. Lab Invest 54:295–303
97. King SB III (1989) Vascular stents and atherosclerosis. Circulation 79:460–462
98. Litvack F (1989) Intravascular stenting for prevention of restenosis: in search of the magic bullet. JACC 13:1092–1093
99. Serruys PW, Strauss BH, Beatt KJ et al. (1991) Angiographic follow-up after placement of a self-expanding coronary stent. New Engl J Med 324:13–17
100. Strauss BH, Serruys PW, de Scheerder IK et al. (1991) A relative risk and analysis of the angiographic predictors of restenosis within the coronary Wallstent. Circulation 84:1636–1643

101. Strauss BH, Serruys PW, Bertrand M et al. (1991) Quantitative angiographic follow-up of the coronary Wallstent in native vessels and bypass grafts (European experience 1986–1990). Am J Cardiol (in press)
102. de Jaegere PP, Serruys PW, Bertrand M et al. (1991) Incidence of restenosis following Wiktor stent implantation for recurrence of stenosis in the first fifty consecutive patients (abstract). Circulation 84 [Abstract Suppl]:A2341
103. Schwartz RS, Murphy JG, Edwards WD, Reither SJ, Vliestra RE, Holmes DR (1990) A practical porcine model of human coronary artery restenosis post PTCA. J Am Coll Cardiol 15:165A
104. Thubikar M, Baker J, Nolan S (1988) Inhibition of atherosclerosis associated with reduction of arterial intramural stress in rabbits. Arteriosclerosis 8:410–418
105. Booth RFG, Martin JF, Honey AC, Hassall DG, Bessley JE, Moncada S (1989) Rapid development of atherosclerotic lesions in the rabbit carotid artery induced by perivascular manipulation. Atherosclerosis 76:257–268
106. Schwartz RS, Murphy JG, Edwards WD, Camrud AR, Vliestra RE, Holmes DR (1991) Restenosis after balloon angioplasty. A practical proliferative model in porcine coronary arteries. Circulation 82:2190–2200
107. Schwartz RS, Huber KC, Edwards WD, Camrud AR, Jorgensen M, Holmes DR (1991) Coronary restenosis and the importance of mutal thrombus: results in a porcine coronary mode (abstract). Circulation [Abstract Suppl] 84:II-71, A283
108. Faxon DP, Weber VJ, Haudenschild C, Gottsman SB, McGovern WA, Ryan TJ (1982) Acute effects of transluminal angioplasty in three experimental models of atherosclerosis. Arteriosclerosis 2:125–133
109. Hoshino T, Yoshida H, Takayama S, Iwase T, Sakata K, Shingu T, Yokoyama S, Mori N, Kaburagi T (1987) Significance of intimal tears in the mechanism of luminal enlargement in percutaneous transluminal coronary angioplasty: correlation of histologic and angiographic findings in postmorten human hearts. Am Heart J 114:503–510
110. Steele PM, Chesebro JH, Stanson AW, Holmes DR, Dewanjee MK, Badimon L, Fuster V (1985) Balloon angioplasty: natural history of the pathophysiological response to injury in a pig model. Circ Res 57:105–112
111. Faxon DP, Sanborn TA, Haudenschild CC (1987) Mechanism of angioplasty and its relation to restensois. Am J Cardiol 60:5B–9B
112. Gerber T, Ge J, Gorge G, Rupprecht HJ, Meyer J (1991) Effect of PTCA on coronary wall architecture analyzed by intravascular ultrasound (abstract). Circulation [Abstract Suppl] 84:A0619
113. Macdonald R, Feldman RL, Conti CR, Pepine CJ (1984) Thromboembolic complications of coronary angioplasty. Am J Cardiol 54:916–917
114. Block PC, Elmer D, Fallon JT (1982) Release of atherosclerotic debris after transluminal angioplasty. Circulation 65:950–952
115. Saber R, Edwards WD, Holmes DR, Vliestra R, Reeder GS (1988) Balloon angioplasty of aortocoronary saphenous vein bypass grafts: a histopathologic study of six grafts from five patients, with emphasis of restenosis and embolic complications. J Am Coll Cardiol 12:1501–1509
116. Garratt KN, Kaufmann UP, Edwards WD, Vliestra RE, Holmes DR (1989) Safety of percutaneous coronary atherectomy with deep arterial resection. Am J Cardiol 64:538–540
117. Kuntz R, Selmon M, Robertson G, Schnitt S, Saflan R. Excision of deep wall components by directional coronary atherectomy does not increase restenosis (abstract). Circulation [Abstract Suppl] 84:A0321
118. Glagov S, Weisenberg E, Zarins CK, Stankunavicius K, Kolettis GJ (1987) Compensatory enlargement of human atherosclerotic coronary arteries. New Engl J Med 316:1371–1375
119. Forrester JS, Eigler N, Litvack F (1991) Interventional cardiology: the decade ahead. Circulation 84:942–944

120. Cook S, Eigler N, Shefer A et al. (1991) Percutaneous excimer laser coronary angioplasty of lesions not favorable for balloon angioplasty. Circulation 84:632–643
121. Ellis SG, DeCasare NB, Pinkerton CA et al. (1991) Relation of stenosis morphology and clinical presentation to the procedural results of directional coronary atherectomy. Circulation 84:644–653
122. Schatz RA, Leon MB, Baim DS, Ellis SG, Erbel R, Hirshfeld JW, Goldberg S, Penn IM (1989) Balloon expandable intracoronary stents: initial results of a multicenter study (abstract). Circulation 80:II-174
123. Nath FC, Muller DW, Ellis SG, Chapekis AT, Zimmerman C, Topol EJ (1991) Early thrombotic occlusion of coronary stents: frequency, predictoes, therapy and clinical outcome (abstract). Circulation [Abstract Suppl] 84:II-587
124. Fischman DL, Savage MP, Leon MB, Hirschfield JW Jr, Cleman MW, Teirstein P, Goldberg S (1991) Angiographic predictors of sub-acute thrombosis following coronary artery stenting (abstract). Circulation [Abstract Suppl]84:II-588
125. Haude M, Swars H, Hopp HW, Franzen D, Heublein B, Meyer J (1991) Subacute thrombotic occlusions as the major complications after intracoronary implantation of Palmaz-Shatz stents: acute management and long-term outcome (abstract). Circulation [Abstract Suppl] 84:II-587
126. Erbel R, Swars H, Hafner G, Haude M, Meyer J (1991) Reduction of subactue thrombotic stent occlusion by improved anticoagulation monitoring (abstract). Circulation [Abstract Suppl] 84:II-588
127. Herman HC, Hirschfield JW Jr, Buchbinder M et al. (1991) Emergent coronary artery stenting for failed PTCA (abstract). Circulation [Abstract Suppl] 84:II-590
128. de Jaegere P, Rensing B, van den Brandt MJ, Suryapranata H (1991) Morphologic change in coronary artery stenosis after stent implantation. Comparison between Wallstent and Wiktor stent (abstract). Circulation 84 [Abstract Suppl]:A0778
129. de Jaegere P, Strauss BH, de Feyter P, Suryapranata H, van den Brand M, Serruys PW (1991) Stent versus balloon angioplasty; matching based on QCA, a surrogate for randomized studies? (abstract). Circulation 84 [Abstract Suppl]:A0782
130. Rensing BJ, Hermans WR, Deckers JW, de Feyter PJ, Tijssen JGP, Serruys PW (1992) Luminal narrowing after percutaneous transluminal coronary balloon angioplasty follows a near Gaussian distribution. A quantitative angiographic study in 1445 successfully dilated lesions. J Am Coll Cardiol 19:939–45
131. Umans VA, Beatt KJ, Rensing BJ, Hermans WR, de Feyter PJ, Serruys PW (1991) Comparative quantitative angiographic analysis of directional coronary atherectomy and balloon angioplasty: a new methodologic approach. Am J Cardiol 1991 68: 1556–1563
132. Hermans WR, Rensing BJ, Kelder JC, de Feyter PJ, Serruys PW (1992) Postangioplasty restenosis rate between segments of the major coronary arteries. Am J Cardiol 69:194–200
133. Meier B (1990) Technique of coronary angioplasty. In: Meier B (ed) Interventional cardiology, Hogrefe and Huber, Toronto, pp 45–69
134. Karsch KR, Haase KK, Voelker W, Bauambach A, Mauser M, Seipel L (1990) Percutaneous coronary excimer laser angioplasty in patients with stable and unstable anginal pectoris: acute results and incidence of restenosis during 6 month follow up. Circulation 81:1849–1859

Bioabsorbable, Drug-Eluting, Intracoronary Stents: Design and Future Applications

R.S. Schwartz,[1] J.G. Murphy,[1] W.D. Edwards,[2] and D.R. Holmes[1]

Introduction

The era of the intracoronary stent has arrived in interventional cardiology. As described elsewhere in this volume, these devices are finding many applications. They frequently permit alternatives to emergency coronary bypass surgery by reestablishing patency of an acutely occluded coronary artery. Long term results with metallic stents are unclear, but appear promising. Stents may find use in maintaining patency and reducing restenosis. Current devices have not been used long enough to assess these issues, nor the issues of long-term side effects.

Intracoronary stents in current use include both balloon-expandable and self-expanding designs [1–9], all of which are metal. These metals are generally spring-tempered stainless steel or elemental tanatalum. Why are these devices made from metals? The physical and mechanical properties of metals make these stents easily deployable using techniques commonly used during PTCA. Excellent radial strength results from both designs in their expanded configuration. The documented ease of deployment, coupled with acceptable tissue biocompatibility represents the initial engineering solution to stent design. Indeed, such designs originated with Dotter's early work in 1969 [10] and current devices have not changed conceptually in over 20 years since this early work.

While there are definite structural and delivery advantages of metallic stents, there are drawbacks as well. Recent advances in biomaterials technology permit consideration of alternative, nonmetallic intracoronary stents. Such devices may allow improved physiologic and clinical results. Because device design typically proceeds through many iterations, it is likely that current metal designs will be considerably modified to overcome current limitations, and additional applications may develop. Current designs likely represent an early phase in an evolutionary course of improved stent designs.

[1] Division of Cardiovascular Diseases, [2] Division of Pathology, Mayo Foundation, 200 1st St SW, Rochester, MN 55905, USA

Coronary Stents
Edited by U. Sigwart and G.I. Frank
© Springer-Verlag Berlin Heidelberg 1992

In this chapter we discuss some design considerations and early work in nonmetallic intracoronary stents, which may lead to improved clinical performance.

Metallic Intracoronary Stents: Advantages and Limitations

The inherent property by which materials recover from mechanical deformation is termed elasticity. The elastic modulus is a parameter used to measure stiffness properties of materials. This modulus, combined with properties of ductility ("formability") determine how "springy" a length of wire will be. The elastic modulus reflects how much that wire can bend before permanent shape changes (plastic deformation) occur. Elastic constants and ductility of many metals may be changed by heat treating (annealing, tempering, quenching, etc.) after forming. The self-expanding Wallstent is made of stainless steel with a resilient temper; it does not maintain a permanent shape change when bent. This stent is helically wound. Following collapse within a delivery catheter, it returns to its initial helical shape when deployed from the catheter. Conversely, balloon-expandable stents are made of stainless steel or tantalum and are designed for plastic deformation. Because of ductility, these stents can be progressively crimped onto a PTCA balloon and expanded in an artery, where they maintain the new, expanded shape.

Ductile and biocompatibility properties make these metals a good compromise for stents, where both reliable delivery and tissue compatibility are essential. These stents are expected to remain in the coronary arteries without chemical or physical degradation for the life of the patients in whom they have been implanted.

Stenting is a useful treatment for acute vessel closure, especially when intimal dissections occur which expose large thrombogenic subintimal surfaces to flowing blood. Despite good soft tissue biocompatibility, stent metals are thrombogenic and are deployed at sites of already active thrombosis. These thrombogenic properties require additional countermeasures such as the infusion of low molecular weight dextran during stent implant [11]. Oral anticoagulation after implant must be given to patients with metallic stents. This need for anticoagulation is one disadvantage of metallic stents, resulting from suboptimal blood compatibility.

The properties which make metal stents easily delivered result in arterial segments which are more rigid than the nearby native artery. This mechanical mismatch may result in higher long-term restenosis and occlusion rates, particularly at the ends of stents. This concept was suggested by investigators studying vascular grafts which are also stiffer than native vessels.

Another disadvantage may be that an indwelling metal device remains in the stented patient for the remainder of his/her life. Given the choice between a chronic device and one which is only temporary, most clinicians would choose the latter. It is unclear whether such arterial segments can be redilated or otherwise revascularized (laser angioplasty, mechanical atherectomy, etc.) with the same success as with native coronary arteries. Bypass grafting may be more difficult in a stented coronary artery segment, especially where multiple contiguous stents have been placed in a vessel.

Metallic stents by themselves will probably not solve the restenosis problem [12]. If stenting could more effectively limit restenosis, greater clinical application would result. Unfortunately, there is evidence [13] that improper stent deployment can *cause* neointimal proliferation. How might the stent be better designed to deal with restenosis? Clinical results indicate that purely mechanical solutions are not likely to have substantial impact. Newer revascularization methods such as mechanical atherectomy, rotary abrasion, laser angioplasty [14], and various heating methods [15] all show restenosis rates similar to conventional dilation. Adjunctive pharmacologic methods will probably be necessary to solve the problem. While metallic stents alone cannot deliver drugs, coatings may permit local, high concentration drug delivery.

Potential Solutions: The Ideal Stent

What would constitute the ideal intracoronary stent? Such a device should be easily deployed and have good fluoroscopic visibility. It should be nonthrombogenic (possibly "antithrombogenic") and temporary, remaining in place only as long as needed to permit adequate arterial healing. It should abolish restenosis, creating instead a thin, smooth, re-endothelialized, fibrocellular conduit of sufficient diameter to permit unimpeded blood flow. Ideally, the natural tissue conduit left by the stent would remain unchanged for the remainder of the patient's life. An ideal stent may not be realizable in practice; the design requirements are quite stringent. Biocompatible polymers have some properties which may provide alternatives to purely metallic devices.

Polymers: A Brief Introduction

Polymers are chemical compounds with many repeating structural subunits; they have substantial medical, industrial, and commercial applications. The chemical industry has synthesized thousands of polymers. Selection of potentially useful polymers for an intracoronary stent draws upon much

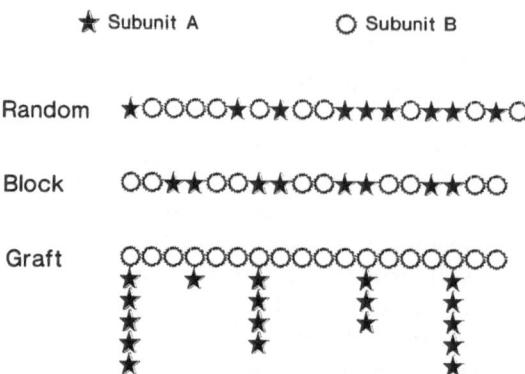

Fig. 1. Schematized examples of hypothetical polymers and nomenclature. Polymers consist of repeating basic subunits in differing combinations. Structures of random, block, and graft polymeric subunit insertion are shown. (Adapted from [16])

industrial research and development. (The vast majority of polymers in medicine today are *not* used for implantable devices, but rather for packaging and in disposable devices such as syringes and intravenous tubing.) Most polymers were initially developed for industrial purposes and later found useful in biomedical applications. This is due to the large costs associated with new polymer research and development.

Different structural patterns of the same repeating polymeric subunits result in materials with quite different mechanical properties. Monomeric polymers (homopolymers) consist of a single repeating basic subunit [16]. More complex polymers can be made with two or more different repeating subunits as shown in Fig. 1. This figure illustrates possible configurations using two schematized subunits. Such a polymer with two repeating subunits is called a copolymer. The biologic behavior of such copolymers differs substantially from the behavior of a homopolymer made solely from either single subunit (monomer). Possible subunit arrangements and consequent biologic properties are unlimited, especially considering that three (terpolymer) or many (multipolymer) subunits can be combined in different configurations.

The biologic behavior of a polymer depends on the repeating subunit configurations, the conformations of the polymerized molecule, and the inter- and intramolecular bonding forces. Polymers frequently exist in forms where polymerized chains of many different lengths make up the macroscopic material. Its properties can be influenced by the range and shape of the molecular weight distribution. Figure 2 shows a hypothetical molecular weight density function which might be typical of any polymer. Low molecular weight portions arise from short chains and usually are waxy or liquid. Additives and reaction residues also contribute to the low molecular

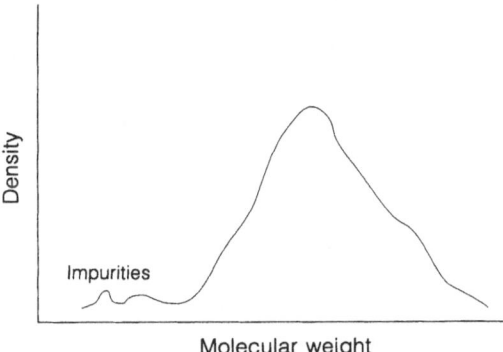

Fig. 2. Distribution of molecular weights in a hypothetical polymer, showing the density distribution function. The variation in molecular weights is due to polymer chains of varying lengths. At the low molecular weight end are the impurities. (Adapted from [16])

Table 1. Chemical structure of common polymers with cardiac application

Polymer name	Structure	Cardiac use
Polyethylene	H H H H H $\mid$ $\mid$ $\mid$ $\mid$ $\mid$ —C—C—C—C—C— $\mid$ $\mid$ $\mid$ $\mid$ $\mid$ H H H H H	Catheters, PTCA balloons
Polytetrafluoroethylene (PTFE, Teflon, Goretex)	F F F F F $\mid$ $\mid$ $\mid$ $\mid$ $\mid$ —C—C—C—C—C— $\mid$ $\mid$ $\mid$ $\mid$ $\mid$ F F F F F	Synthetic grafts, catheters
Polypropylene (Prolene)	H CH$_3$ H H $\mid$ $\mid$ $\mid$ $\mid$ —C—C—C—C— $\mid$ $\mid$ $\mid$ $\mid$ H H H CH$_3$	Vascular suture
Polyethylene terephthalate (Dacron, Mylar)	H H O H H O $\mid$ $\mid$ $\parallel$ C—C $\parallel$ —O—C—C—O—C—C C—C— $\mid$ $\mid$ C=C H H H H	PTCA balloons
Polyurethane	O O $\parallel$ $\parallel$ —C—N—(CH$_2$)$_2$—N—C—O—(CH$_2$)$_2$— $\mid$ $\mid$ H H	Pacing leads

weight content of polymers. The higher molecular weight portions arise from long chains and usually are harder and less flexible.

Polymeric blood compatibility is dominated by the outermost molecular layers in blood contact. The polymer surface is thus critical for blood contact applications. In some polymers, surface characteristics are quite different from those of the bulk polymer just a few molecular layers deeper. Agents used to synthesize the polymer or give it desirable physical features such as flexibility (plasticizing agents) frequently migrate to the polymer surface, resulting in altered biocompatibility. Much study is thus concentrating on polymer surface properties and their modification. Certain additives incorporated during polymer synthesis result in novel, potentially beneficial biologic surface properties. These additives are called surface modifying additive (SMA) substances. SMA substances migrate to the polymer surface after synthesis, and may provide a useful compromise between desirable surface and bulk polymer properties. The polymeric intracoronary stent will need suitable bulk properties for practical intracoronary delivery. It will also require excellent surface properties to prevent thrombosis and to avoid stimulation of neointimal hyperplasia. Surface modifying technology may helpful in satisfying both of these needs.

Typical polymers used for biomedical devices today exhibit good tissue compatibility (Table 1). They also provide adequate mechanical strength. These polymers are biostable and do not degrade signficantly over time within the body. They also cannot deliver drugs easily. While they are termed biocompatible, they still are somewhat thrombogenic.

Thrombogenicity of Polymers and Other Foreign Materials

Thrombosis and coagulation are powerful survival mechanisms in all higher animal species. Blood normally clots only at sites of vascular injury, yet remains fluid elsewhere in the body. Endothelial cells, continuous throughout the vascular tree, are critical for regulating the delicate balance between fluid and clotted blood. The endothelium as described by Virchow was historically considered an inert cell layer. He postulated that endothelial violation exposed thrombogenic subintima, activating protective clotting mechanisms. He viewed the endothelium as a passive protective lining. Recent evidence reveals the endothelial cell is far from inert. It synthesizes a variety of antithrombotic substances including von Willebrand's factor, t-PA, urokinase, prostacyclin, and thrombomodulin, which collectively enable low local thrombogenic potential. The normal homeostatic coagulation milieu may thus be a highly active equilibrium process modulated by endothelium. Endothelial surfaces continually neutralize thrombin and lyse fibrin. This finding has significant impact for polymeric stents within arteries. Foreign surfaces may be recognized as such by blood if key substances are *not* actively elaborated. A nonthrombogenic manmade material may not be possible, at least in passive form. Some investigators have considered seeding foreign arterial implants with endothelial cells to help overcome problems of passive material surfaces [17–19].

An understanding of coagulation is critical to polymeric intracoronary stent design. Studies of foreign surface/blood interfaces indicate the importance of surface electric charge [20, 21], thermodynamic surface energy and chemistry[1] [22], and surface texture. These studies may have oversimplified the interactions. For example, it was thought that materials with net negative surface charge (negative electrochemical potentials) are highly blood compatible. After rigorous testing however, this hypothesis may be an erroneous simplification. There are no simple rules governing interactions between blood and foreign materials.

The interaction between blood and polymers is initiated by the attachment of plasma proteins [23]. Such proteins are usually fibrinogen and fibrin [24], constituting a conditioning film. This film initiates a second phase of biologic interaction, platelet adhesion and aggregation. Complement activation by C3 and C5 also occurs early in foreign material-blood interactions. Following platelet adhesion and aggregation, activation of the extrinsic clotting system by damaged tissue completes the clotting process [25].

Polymeric blood compatibility relates to which specific plasma proteins deposit on the implanted material. Many passive foreign surfaces become coated with albumin (as in some artificial organs), which may be beneficial. Fibrin may attach to those foreign bodies which are less blood compatible. Currently, many problems remain; there is no truly blood-compatible foreign material [26–28].

An important distinction should be made between materials which are *blood compatible* and those which are *biocompatible* (soft-tissue compatible). Materials which are blood compatible are biocompatible, but the converse is not always true since blood compatibility requirements are much more stringent. Little is known about blood compatibility of many polymers, and no universally accepted evaluation standards exist.

One problem concerning polymeric blood compatibility is the multiplicity of evaluation techniques available. Four basic types of tests are used:

1. In vitro tests: Polymers are exposed to blood elements in a benchtop setting outside a vascular space. One advantage of this test is low cost. However, the applicability of test results to in vivo situations is uncertain. Misleading results are frequently obtained.

---

[1] One estimate of the surface energy in a polymer is to measure the angle formed between the surface and a bead of water placed on that surface: The more hydrophobic, the larger the surface free energy and, some believe, the more blood compatible.

2. Extracorporeal tests: Blood flows directly from a cannulated animal artery into a test chamber containing the polymer of interest. Interactions can be monitored in detail. Protein absorption and platelet reaction studies are usually performed in this manner.

3. Tubular devices in animals: The polymer of interest is formed into a cylinder and implanted in an animal artery. This method is more expensive, and results depend on variables such as flow, artery size, and other local hemodynamics. These variables can unknowingly bias results.

4. Membrane fabrication: The polymer is formed into a thin membrane and put into a flow chamber. Downstream blood samples are studied for hemolysis or complement activation.

Useful Polymer Characteristics: Bioabsorbability and Drug Elution

Biostable polymers such as polypropylene vascular sutures remain intact after placement for many years. Theoretical advantages of an intracoronary stent made from such biostable materials are uncertain; one improvement might be lower thrombogenicity.

An alternative approach to biostable materials is a bioabsorbable stent, remaining intact for a pre-determined time while gradually dissolving. Bioabsorbable (also referred to as bioerodable or biodegradable) polymers generally disintegrate by chemical hydrolysis. Three hydrolytic mechanisms are known. In the first, long chain polymers connected by hydrolyzable cross linkages separate when the crosslinks are hydrolyzed. Other polymers are water insoluble but easily hydrolyze to soluble products which may be carried away by body fluids. These solubilization products are frequently large molecules, not easily eliminated via the kidney or liver. Polymers used systemically which erode via this mechanism are problematic. They are thus used principally in topical applications. In the third disintegration mechanism, insoluble polymers with labile backbones (Fig. 1) are split through hydrolysis of that backbone. The resulting products are low molecular weight and water soluble, making these polymers most suitable for systemic uses. Many polymers erode through combinations of hydrolytic mechanisms.

Polymer degradation has two types of macroscopic behavior, homogeneous and heterogeneous. Heterogeneous degradation occurs at the polymer surface only. Gross structural integrity of the polymer remains, much like ice melting in a glass of warm water. Homogeneous degradation, by comparison, occurs evenly throughout the structure. This causes fragmentation and structural integrity loss soon after implantation, much like the piecemeal breakup of an iceberg. Most bioabsorbable polymers degrade via both mechanisms. More hydrophobic polymers tend toward heterogeneous mechanisms and hydrophilic polymers toward homogeneous dissolution through hydration. Fragmentation of an absorbable polymeric stent could have adverse effects if gross embolization occurred. If the polymer maintains its structural integrity for more than a few weeks, concerns for embolization may be unnecessary since thrombus and neointima would likely cover the device.

Degradation times can be as short as a few hours or as long as many years, even for the same polymer. Degradation times depend on bulk polymer configuration, additives, and fabrication methods. Through changes in synthetic methods, polymers can be programmed for different degradation rates. This property is a definite advantage to their potential use in intra-coronary stenting. It is thus important to establish how long a coronary stent must remain in place.

Biodegradability provides a means for controlled release of incorporated drugs [29–31]. This scheme permits continuous, concentrated, local elution of desired bioactive agents. High local concentrations could translate into low systemic doses which would be well tolerated. All polymer and drug would disappear at the end of the programmed degradation time [32]. This concept provides potential solutions to the two major problems in PTCA today: acute vessel closure and long-term restenosis. First, the macroscopic configuration of the polymeric stent could maintain the dilated state of the vessel and also support intimal dissections. Second, as yet undefined pharmacologic agents which limit intimal hyperplasia could be incorporated directly into such a stent. Antithrombotic agents might also be incorporated into the polymer matrix to reduce local thrombosis at the dilated site.

A few bioabsorbable polymers are well suited for drug impregnation and delivery during polymer degradation. Polymers degrading through the backbone hydrolysis mechanism will likely be most useful for the intra-coronary stent[2]. Some of these polymers are in use for intramuscular, intraperitoneal, and subcutaneous drug delivery systems. Table 2 lists some candidate bioabsorbable polymers for coronary stent applications. The most promising of these are discussed below.

Polylactic Acid, Polyglycolic Acid Copolymers

These polymers are polyesters [33–35]. They have been studied most com-prehensively of all degradable and drug-eluting polymers. Their first use was in absorbable sutures during the early 1970s. PLA/PGA erodes relatively homogeneously to lactic acid, glycolic acid, water, and carbon dioxide. These degradation products have little toxicity but do generate an inflam-matory response. These polymers have been considered for implantable,

---

[2] Polymers degrading through crosslink hydrolysis are most readily combined with drugs of low water solubility and thus of limited use in the bloodstream.

Table 2. Bioabsorbable polymers with possible stent applications

---

Polylactic acid/polyglycolic acid
Polyanhydrides
Polyorthoesters
Polyphosphate esters
Polyiminocarbonates
Polyurethanes (absorbable)
Polyhydroxybutyrates
Polycaprolactones
Polytrimethylene carbonates

---

long-acting contraceptives. One problem our group encountered in using extruded thin, extruded PLA/PGA fibers was brittleness resulting in the inability to make tight bends without fracture. Such fibers must be formed into a stent and mounted in a delivery system, later to expand into a supportive stent form. Plasticizers or other synthetic methods may result in better PLA/PGA physical properties. Little has been published regarding blood compatibility of PLA/PGA. Vessel inflammation at the implant site remains a theoretical concern. Drug loading of this polymer is also more difficult.

The *polyanhydrides* [36] were discovered early in this century. They underwent extensive study in the late 1950s, when they were under consideration as replacements for polyester fibers. They were discarded due to their hydrolyzability. The polyanhydrides erode heterogenously, typically through surface erosion. They exhibit good tissue biocompatibility and minimal degradation product toxicity [37–39]. Rare inflammation and mild fibrosis resulted when implanted subcutaneously in rats. Exposure of these polymers to ultrasonic energy may be a means of modulating drug release. Current clinical applications include local delivery of chemotherapeutic agents active against central nervous system malignancies. These polymers will require blood compatibility studies prior to use in stents.

The *polyorthoesters* are another biodegradable polymer group which hydrolyze rapidly in acid but are more slowly hydrolyzed in alkaline media. These compounds are in clinical tests for releasing contraceptive steroids within subcutaneous implants. They undergo heterogeneous degradation. Incorporated drugs may form small "bubbles" within the polymer during manufacture. During hydration, the polymer swells, and adjacent bubbles are connected. Eventually the bubbles become confluent with the polymer surface causing drug release. A skeleton of absorbable bulk polymer remains after all drug is gone. The polymer skeleton usually erodes more slowly than the time required for drug release. Through compositional and fabrication manipulations, constant drug release can be obtained.

The *polyiminocarbonates* [40] are also potential polymers for the biodegradable, drug-eluting, intracoronary stent. These compounds have not been used in medical or industrial applications. The polyiminocarbonates are hydrolyzed either by acid or basic media. They degrade to carbon dioxide, ammonia, and alcohols or phenols related to the original polymer makeup. Little toxicity has been found from initial work with these substances. Subcutaneous mouse implants revealed little inflammatory reaction. Their mechanical properties may permit use as an intracoronary stent.

The *polyphosphate esters* are an interesting, new group of polymers which show promise for formability into mechanically useful stent configurations. They are bioabsorbable and capable of eluting drugs. Such drugs can reportedly be proteins. Another adavantage to this family of polymers is that their degradation time can be readily changed by varying the composition.

Experimentation on pharmacologic agents which may be incorporated into bioabsorbable polymers is expanding. Previously, only drugs of relative molecular weight 600 or less were usable, but more recently these limitations have been overcome. Small proteins can now be incorporated for slow release in some classes of polymers. Polymers capable of delivering proteins may be quite useful, as many growth factors and other vasoactive substances are proteins.

Little has been published about development of bioabsorbable, drug-eluting, intracoronary stents, likely because of the newness of this concept. Polymer implantation at angioplasty sites has been proposed in the form of "polymeric endoluminal paving" [41]. In this method, a polymer is heat formed at the arterial delivery site. Few in vivo results have been published about this method.

Research into biodegradable stents is proceeding in parallel with research into the pathophysiology of restenosis. When the etiology of restenosis is better defined, more effective pharmacologic targeting should be possible. Local, chronic, high concentrations of one or more drugs delivered by polymer may better approach this difficult clinical problem.

Materials Evaluation: The Problem of Neointimal Hyperplasia

Luminal obstruction by neointimal hyperplasia is a severe clinical problem in both the native circulation and synthetic vascular grafts [42]. Routine success has not been achieved in synthetic grafts of less than 6 mm, since smaller grafts develop occlusive proliferative neointima. This neointima typically emanates from anastamotic sites, eventually causing prosthetic thrombosis. Similarly, late restenosis after coronary angioplasty is caused by neointimal proliferation. Histopathologically, the neointima in each of these situations has many common properties. Smooth muscle cell derived myofibroplasia is frequently seen in conjunction with intercellular ground substance. Figure 3 shows a high power microscopic view of the neointima

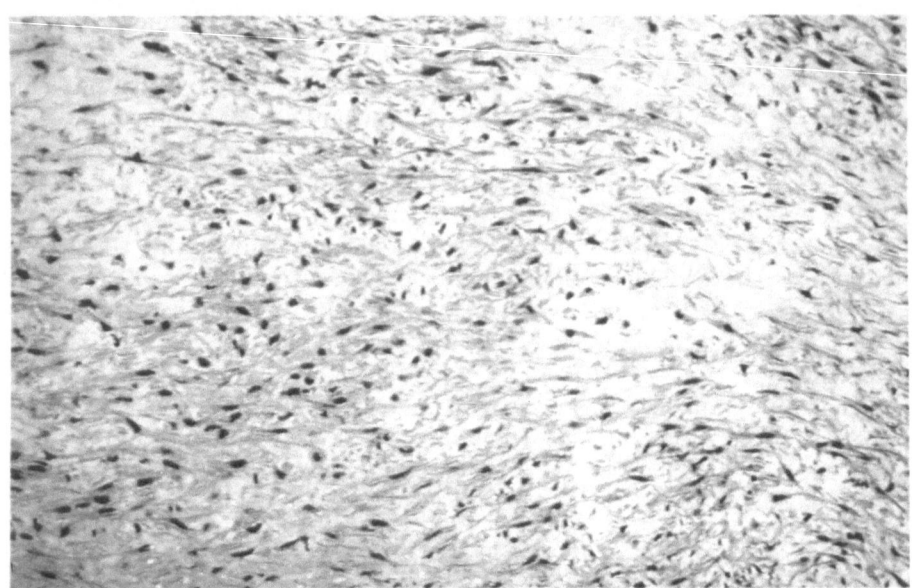

Fig. 3. Photomicrograph of neointimal hyperplasia from a human restenotic lesion 3 months after PTCA. Elastic van Gieson stain, x30

from human restenosis following PTCA. The histopathologic similarities between these processes suggest that arteries respond both to injury and foreign bodies in similar ways, although the mechanisms are not well understood.

The ideal polymeric stent and bioactive agent should promote organized neointimal growth to a point and then cease. This would result in a patent, endothelialized, biologic lumen for flowing blood. Toward this end, the elucidation of neointimal pathophysiology and control will be an achievement of major clinical proportions. Resolution of restenosis, longer synthetic vascular graft lifetimes, and successful smaller diameter synthetic grafts would result. Coronary bypass with synthetic grafts would be possible.

A porcine model of intense coronary arterial neointimal proliferation has been recently developed in our laboratory [13] to help understand restenosis pathophysiology. Severe injury to normal pig coronary arteries results from implanting grossly oversized metallic coils. Within 28 days of injury, the proliferative neointima resulting from this injury identically duplicates the tissue responsible for human restenosis. This model may also be useful for testing polymer blood compatibility prior to intracoronary stent construction. Figure 4 shows neointimal hyperplasia in a pig coronary artery injured by this metallic coil method. This tissue consists of cells derived from medial smooth muscle, loosely embedded in intercellular ground substance. This histopathologic makeup differs sharply from atherosclerotic plaque.

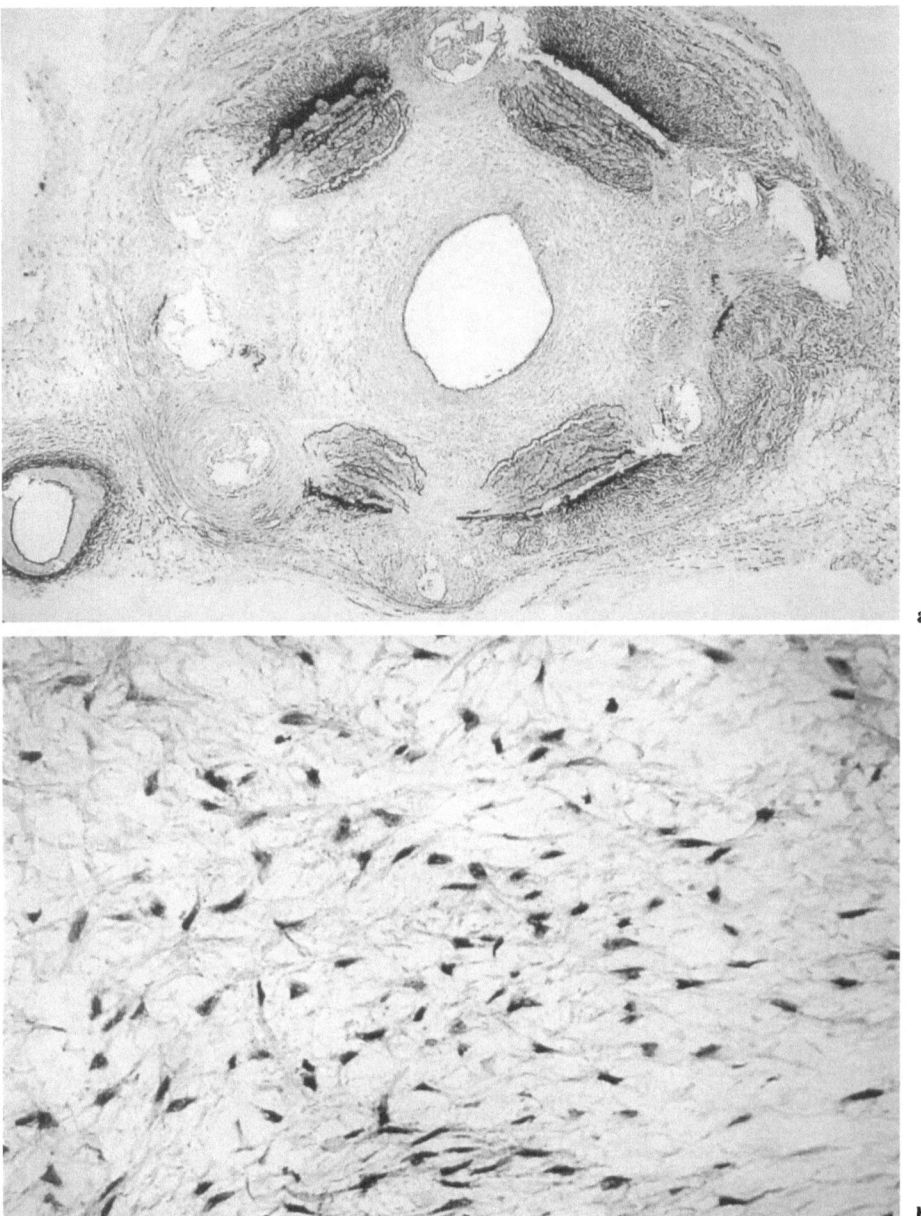

Fig. 4. a Severe neointimal hyperplasia induced by metallic coil injury to a normal pig artery. The small circumferential holes are where the wires were located. The hole in the center is the residual lumen, severely compromised by proliferative neointima. This proliferative neointima is identical to the proliferative neointima found in human restenosis. **b** The proliferative neointima at higher magnification. The intercellular ground substance is loose. These cells stain strongly for actin, suggesting that they derive from media, of smooth muscle origin. This neointima also bears striking resemblance to the neointima of prosthetic arterial grafts

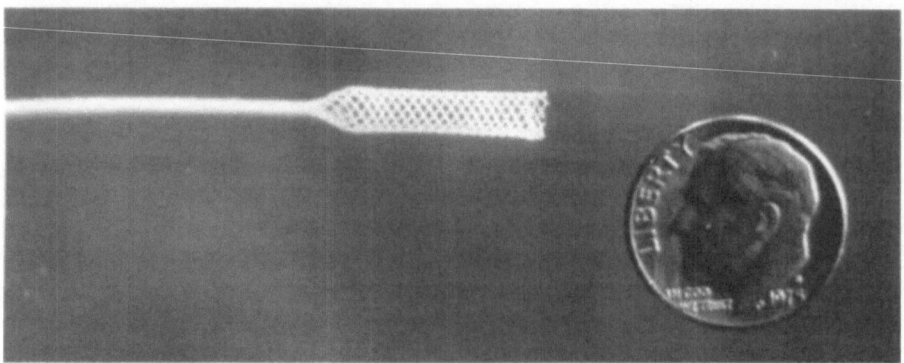

Fig. 5. The self-expanding, biostable, polyethylene terephthalate (PET) stent and delivery catheter

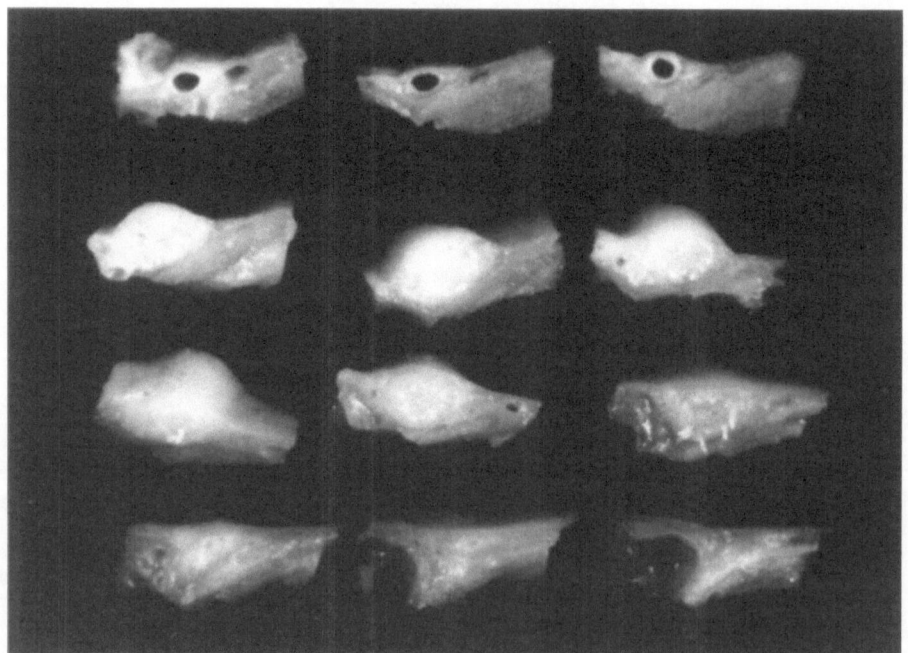

Fig. 6. a Total occlusion resulted after 4 weeks of PET stent implant in a porcine left anterior descending coronary artery. Sequential arterial cross sections are shown from the same artery, proceeding through the stent. **b** Low power photomicrograph of the polymeric stent result. Holes are from the PET strands. Darker areas indicate inflammation and foreign body reaction by the artery. **c** Neointima shown at high power from the PET stent experiment. Note the smooth muscle cell nuclei, similar ground substance, and a giant cell in the center of the picture, indicating the foreign body reaction

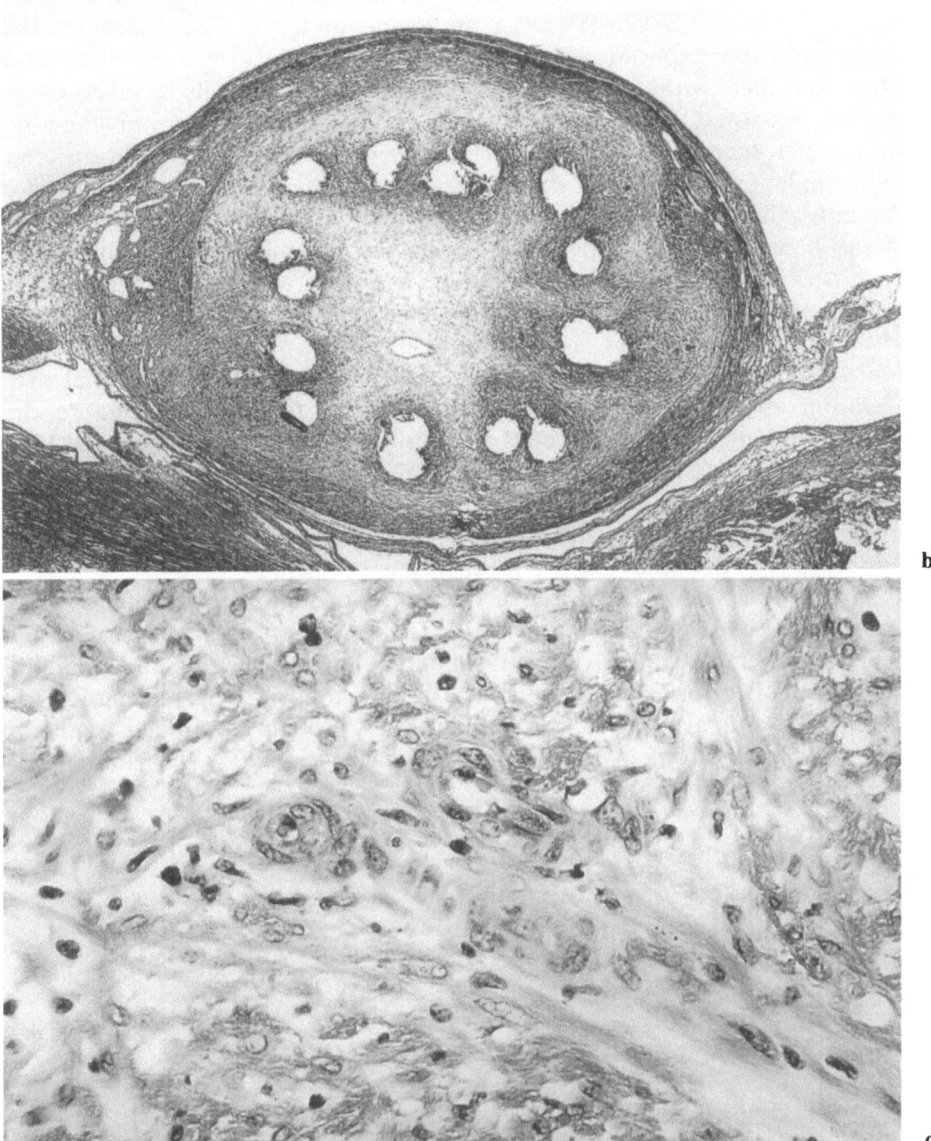

Fig. 6. Continued

As a pilot study of polymeric stent configurations and blood compatibility, polyethylene terephthalate (PET) strands (0.006″, 0.15 mm) were woven into the dual counter-helical stent design shown in Fig. 5. PET is biostable, with an estimated survival in the body of more than 30 years. This configuration is self-expanding after release from the custom-designed delivery catheter. Seven Yucatan miniswine underwent coronary arterial implant of these experimental PET stents. The animals were fed a standard laboratory diet, without lipid supplementation. The animals received intra-arterial heparin (10000-unit bolus) at the time of implant only and no antiplatelet agents. All pigs were clinically well for the entire period after stent implant (range 29–41 days), except one which died acutely 2 h after implant. After the animals were killed, gross and microscopic examination of the hearts was performed. All hearts showed myocardial infarction in the distribution of the stent-implanted coronary artery. Coronary artery examination revealed total occlusion in all animals, as shown in Fig. 6a. Microscopic examination showed areas of severe neointimal hyperplasia, associated with organizing thrombus. An example of the neointimal proliferation under higher power is shown in Fig. 6b,c. In addition to the neointimal hyperplasia, giant cells and eosinophils were noted near the PET stent struts, consistent with a mild foreign body response. It is likely that thrombus deposition occurred on this biostable polymeric stent, associated with the severe neointimal proliferation. The relation of the hyperplasia to thrombus is under study, as are mechanisms to decrease each.

In the pig, acute occlusion of one or more major epicardial coronary arteries causes acute ischemic death. The pig heart is similar to human hearts in lacking a well developed collateral circulation. Only one animal in this small pilot series died suddenly, despite total coronary occlusions in all chronic animals. These coronary arteries probably occluded gradually and completely from progressive neointimal thickening. This finding was

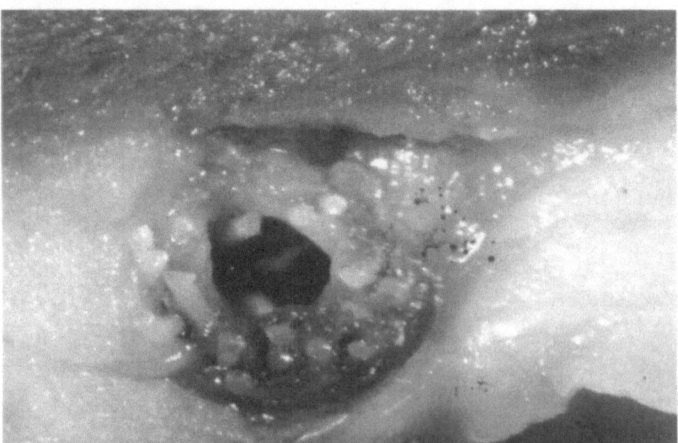

Fig. 7. Gross photographic cross section of a pig in which the polymeric PET stent was implanted in an identical manner as in Fig. 6. In this case, however, the animal received daily oral aspirin, and the vessel remained patent although the stent strands are covered by neointima similar to that seen in Fig. 6

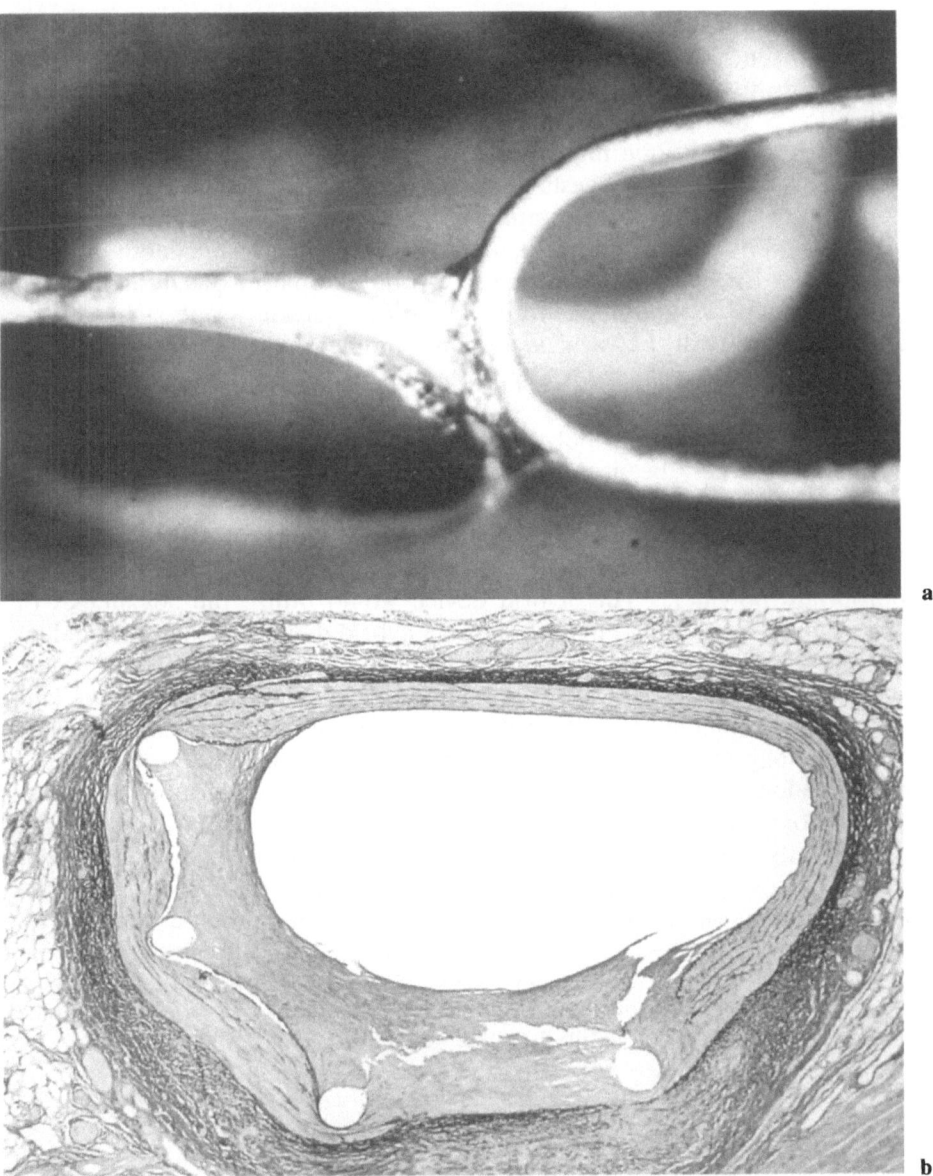

a

b

Fig. 8. a Closeup view of a hybrid tantalum coil coated with polyphosphate ester, 0.001″ (0.025 mm) thick. The metal coil is 0.005″ (0.125 mm). This device is shown prior to implant in a pig coronary artery. **b** Low power photomicrograph of a representative pig coronary artery in which the hybrid tantalum/polyphosphate ester coil was implanted for 28 days. All polymer had degraded, and there was no histopatholgic evidence of toxicity or foreign body response

unexpected and calls into question the long-term blood compatibility of PET without adjunctive pharmacologic therapy. The small coronary artery diameter of the pig (2.0–3.0 mm) is a more realistic test for eventual human application than a larger peripheral arterial implant. Toward this end, daily oral aspirin given in one pig resulted in good patency, as shown grossly in Fig. 7. This experience suggests the importance of platelets in the genesis of neointima. Further experimentation with PET using other pharmacologic agents, as well as with other polymers, is proceeding in our laboratory. If the proliferative hyperplastic response can be pharmacologically modulated to stop under an endothelialized cylindrical polymer, one goal of the idealized stent will be achieved. This problem exemplifies difficulties encountered in the search for appropriate blood compatible materials. The pig model may prove useful for testing in vivo blood compatibility of bioabsorbable drug eluting polymers. Initially, experience with biostable polymers will likely be useful for the subsequent design of bioabsorbable devices.

If total absorbability and drug-elution requirements prove too stringent, a compromise might be reached by coating current metallic stents with appropriate polymers. This hybrid device would utilize the advantages of each group of materials. Figure 8 shows a hybrid device in which a tantalum coil was totally imbedded in a layer of polyphosphate ester (0.001″ thick, 0.025 mm). These devices were implanted in the coronary arteries of four pigs, and all remained patent until the animals were killed at 28 days. The histopathology from these animals was little different than from the coil implants alone, showing no evidence of toxicity or foreign body reaction. Furthermore, the polymer had successfully degraded from these stents, leaving only bare tantalum wire. Such hybrid devices are also under evaluation to establish the compatibility of polymers, as are a number of pharmacologic agents which could be delivered through such a stent.

Acknowledgements. We would like to express thanks for expert technical advice to Messrs. Rod Wolff and Vince Hull of Medtronic, Inc., and to Dr. Arthur Coury (Medtronic, Inc.) for review of this manuscript.

References

1. Sigwart U, Puel J, Mirkovitch V, Joffre F, Kappenberger L (1987) Intravascular stents to prevent occlusion and restenosis after transluminal angioplasty. N Engl J Med 316(12):701–706
2. Sigwart U, Urban P, Golf S, Kaufmann U, Imbert C, Fischer A, Kappenberger L (1988) Emergency stenting for acute occlusion after coronary balloon angioplasty. Circulation 78(5):1121–1127
3. Ellis S, Topol E (1989) Intracoronary stents: will they fulfill their promise as an adjunct to angioplasty? J Am Coll Cardiol 13(6):1425–1430

4. Schatz R, Palmaz J, Tio F, Garcia F, Garcia O, Reuter S (1987) Balloon expandable intracoronary stents in the adult dog. Circulation 76:450–456
5. Wright K, Wallace S, Charnsangavij C, Carrasco C, Gianturco C (1985) Percutaneous endovascular stents: an experimental evaluation. Radiology 156:261
6. Roubin G, Robinson K, King SB III, Gianturco C, Bloch AJ, Brown J, Siegel R, Douglas J (1987) Early and late results of intracoronary arterial stenting after coronary angioplasty in dogs. Circulation 76:450–456
7. White C, Ramee S, Banks A, Ross T, Wiktor D, Chokshi S, Price H, Isner J (1990) Angiographic patency of a tantalum coil stent (abstract). J Am Coll Cardiol 15(2): 119A
8. Fishman D, Savage M, Leon M, Hirshfeld J, Cleman M, Ellis S, Schatz R, Goldberg S (1990) Effect of intracoronary stenting on intimal dissection following balloon angioplasty: results of qualitative and quantitative coronary analysis (abstract). J Am Coll Cardiol 15(2):119A
9. Schatz R, Leon M, Baim D, Ellis S, Marco J, Erbel R, Goldberg S (1990) Short-term results and complications with the Palmaz-Schatz coronary stent (abstract). J Am Coll Cardiol 15(2):119A
10. Dotter C (1969) Transluminally placed coilspring endoarterial tube grafts. Long term patency in canine popliteal artery. Invest Radiol 4:327–332
11. Palmaz J, Garcia O, Copp D (1987) Balloon expandable intra-arterial stents: effect of anticoagulation on thrombus formation (abstract). Circulation 76 [Suppl IV]:IV–45
12. Sutton C, Kambic H, Oku T, Harasaki H, Imoto H, Tominaga R, Hollman J (1988) Stenting fails to prevent recurrent stenosis in the rabbit model of atherosclerosis (abstract). Circulation 78 [Suppl II]:II–414
13. Schwartz R, Murphy J, Edwards W, Camrud A, Vlietstra R, Holmes D (1990) Restenosis after balloon angioplasty: a practical proliferative model in porcine coronary arteries. Circulation 82:2190–2200
14. Sanborn T, Hershman R, Siegel R, Schatz R, Schnee M, Leachman D, Bittl J (1990) Percutaneous coronary excimer laser-assisted balloon angioplasty: initial multicenter experience (abstract). J Am Coll Cardiol 15(2):25A
15. Ferguson J, Dear W, Leatherman L, Safian R, King S, Douglas J, Spears J (1990) A multi-center trial of laser balloon angioplasty for abrupt closure following PTCA. J Am Coll Cardiol 15(2):25A
16. Ward R (1989) Surface modifying additives for biomedical polymers. IEEE Eng Med Biol 2(8):22–25
17. Graham LM, Vinter DW, Ford JW, Kahn RH, Burker WE, Stanley JC (1980) Endothelial Cell Seeding of Prosthetic vascular grafts. Arch Surg 115:929–933
18. Herring MB, Compton R, Legrand DR, Gardner AL (1989) Endothelial cell seeding in the management of vascular thrombosis. Semin Thromb Hemost 15(2):200–205
19. Van der Giessen WJ, Serruys PW, Visser W, Verdouin PD, van Schalkwijk WP, Jongkind JF (1989) Endothelialization of intravascular stents. J Interven Cardiol 1:109–120
20. Baier R (1972) Role of surface energy in thrombogenesis. Bull NY Acad Sci 48:235
21. De Palma V, Baier R, Ford J, Gott V, Furusse A (1972) Investigation of three surface properties of several metals and their relation to blood compatibility. J Biomed Mater Res Sym 3:137
22. Sawyer PN, Srinivasan S Role of electrochemical surface properties in thrombosis at vascular interfaces. Bull NY Acad Sci 48:235
23. Williams D, Gaskill I, Smith R (1972) Protein Absorption and desorption phenomenon on clean metal surfaces. J Biomed Mater Res 19:313–320
24. Andrade J, Hlady V Plasma protein adsorption: the big twelve. In: Leonard EF, Turitto VT, Vroman L (eds) Blood in contact with natural and artificial surfaces. NY Acad Sci 516:158–172
25. Colman RW, Scott C, Schmaier A, Wachtfogel Y, Pixley R, Edmunds L Initiation of Blood coagulation at artificial surfaces. In: Leonard EF, Turitto VT, Vroman L (eds) Blood in contact with natural and artificial surfaces. NY Acad Sci 516:253–267

26. Coleman DL, King RN, Andrade JD (1974) The foreign body reaction: a chronic inflammatory response. J Biomed Mater Res 8:199
27. Hench LL, Ethridge ED (1982) Biomaterials: an interfacial approach. Academic, New York, Chap 6
28. Greisler HP (1990) Interactions at the blood/material interface. Ann Vasc Surg 4(1):98–103
29. Langer R, Lund D, Leong K, Folkman J (1985) Controlled release of macromolecules: biological studies. J Contr Release 2:331–341
30. Langer RS, Peppas NA (1981) Present and future applications of biomaterials in controlled drug delivery systems. Biomaterials 2:201
31. Heller J (1980) Controlled release of biologically active compounds from bioerodible polymers. Biomaterials 1:51
32. Rosen H, Kohn J, Leong K, Langer R Bioerodible polymers for controlled release systems. In: Hsieh DST (ed) Controlled release systems: fabrication technology. CRC Press, Boca Raton
33. Wise DL, Fellmann TD, Sanderson JE, Wentworth RL (1979) Lactic/glycolic acid polymers. In: Gregoriadis G (ed) Drug carriers in biology and medicine. Academic, London, p 237
34. Gilding DK, Reed AM (1979) Biodegradable polymers for use in surgery-polyglycolic/polylactic acid homo- and copolymers. Polymer 20:1459
35. Morgan MN (1969) New synthetic absorbable suture material. Br Med J 2:308
36. Bucher JE, Slade WC (1909) The anhydrides of isophthalic and terephthalic acids. J Am Chem Soc 31:1319
37. Rosen HB, Chang J, Wnek GE, Linhardt RJ, Langer R (1983) Bioerodible polyanhydrides for controlled drug delivery. Biomaterials 3:141
38. Leong KW, Brott BC, Langer R (1985) Bioerodible polyanhydrides as drug-carrier matrices. I Characterization, degradation, and release characteristics. J Biomater Res 19:941–955
39. Leong KW, D'Amore P, Marletta M, Langer R (1986) Bioerodible polyanhydrides as drug-carrier matrices. II. Biocompatibility and chemical reactivity. J Biomed Mater Res 20:51–64
40. Kohn J, Langer R (1986) Poly (iminocarbonates) as potential biomaterials. Biomaterials 7:176–182
41. Slepian M, Schindler A (1988) Polymeric endoluminal paving and sealing: a biodegradable alternative to intracoronary stenting (abstract). Circulation 78 [Suppl IV]: II-409
42. Malone JM, Reinert RL, Brendel K, Duhamel RC (1984) Thrombogenicity of small diameter vascular grafts. Trans Soc Biomater 3:339

Bioabsorbable Endovascular Stent Prostheses

R.S. Gammon, G.D. Chapman, R.P. Bauman, and R.S. Stack[1]

Introduction

Atherosclerotic cardiovascular disease remains the leading cause of death in industrialized countries. Medical treatment has been largely unsuccessful in altering its course. Surgery is an effective treatment in selected cases but carries with it significant morbidity. Percutaneous balloon angioplasty has been developed as an alternative treatment. Since its introduction by Dotter [1] in peripheral arteries, and Grüntzig [2] in coronary arteries, angioplasty has seen a dramatic rise in popularity. In the USA alone, over 200 000 coronary angioplasties will be performed in 1990 [3]. However, the success of PTCA has been limited by two major complications: acute vessel closure and late restenosis.

Excessive vessel distention required to deform plaque consistently results in some degree of intimal disruption during PTCA [4]. In approximately 5% of cases, intimal dissection results in an obstructive flap, and this, along with abrupt thrombus formation, results in acute vessel occlusion [5]. Repeated, prolonged dilatations, in conjunction with thrombolytic therapy, restore vessel patency in some instances. Despite these efforts, 3%–4% of patients undergoing PTCA will require emergent coronary artery bypass grafting [6, 7].

After more than 10 years experience with balloon angioplasty in coronary arteries, the incidence of restenosis remains unchanged. Some 30%–42% of patients undergoing the procedure will have recurrence of a significant stenosis [8–15]. The pathogenesis of the restenosis process involves a complex interaction between endothelial cells, smooth muscle cells, platelets, monocytes, and lipoproteins [8]. Plaque disruption results in local rheologic alterations such as turbulent flow and shear stress which may contribute to the restenosis process [14]. Platelets adhering to the denuded area release mitogenic factors such as platelet derived growth factor which stimulate local cell replication. Intimal disruption exposes smooth muscle cells to the shear stress of arterial blood flow and this, plus stretch injury of

[1] Interventional Cardiac Catheterization Research Program, Biomedical Engineering Research Department, Duke University Medical Center, Durham, NC 27710, USA

Coronary Stents
Edited by U. Sigwart and G.I. Frank
© Springer-Verlag Berlin Heidelberg 1992

these cells [16], may stimulate release of other factors important in the restenosis process.

Late restenosis appears to be independent of technique or operator skill. Alterations in inflation pressures [17] and durations [18], laser balloon angioplasty [19], and even transluminal surgical excision [20–23] have all failed to reduce restenosis significantly. Numerous pharmacologic agents have been tried without consistent success [24–35]. A number of agents with potential impact on restenosis remain untested because systemic therapy is not practical. Other agents that are ineffective at reducing restenosis when given systemically may be effective if applied locally in high concentration. A means of sustained, local drug delivery precisely at the site of angioplasty is needed.

Endovascular stents address both the problem of acute occlusion [36, 37] and late restenosis [38]. Intimal flaps are tacked to the vessel wall by the scaffolding provided by the stent, restoring flow after an occlusion and reducing smooth muscle cell exposure. The improved luminal geometry [39, 40] establishes a laminar flow pattern which further reduces smooth muscle cell trauma and discourages thrombus formation. The outward radial force provided by the stent resists vasospasm at the site of angioplasty. In addition, the physical presence of the stent might prevent a recurrent lesion from encroaching on the vessel lumen, forcing it to expand outwardly [41].

The purpose of this chapter is to review the development of the Duke bioabsorbable stent [42] that was designed to address the mechanical complications of angioplasty without being a permanent implant. In addition, these devices lend themselves favorably to use for drug delivery by acting as a drug depot. Metallic stents may decrease, but not eliminate, restenosis [43, 44]. However, a bioabsorbable prosthesis, acting as a mechanical stent and drug depot, might accomplish this.

Finally, bioabsorbable stents could provide a means for local delivery of endothelial cells which have been genetically altered to produce a variety of substances (e.g., tissue plasminogen activator). These endothelial cells could be incorporated into a bioabsorbable stent and, once implanted, could result in rapid endothelialization and local drug delivery.

Table 1. Limitations of metallic stents

Limited flexibility
Compliance mismatch
Thrombosis
Intimal hyperplasia/restenosis
Vessel wall (media) thinning
Vasospasm
Incomplete expansion
Balloon rupture
Migration and embolization
Metallic corrosion/toxicity
Permanent foreign body

Limitations of Current Stent Prototypes

Despite the theoretical attractiveness of stents, many concerns must be addressed. All stent prototypes currently available are metallic. While easily performing the mechanical function required, metallic stents still have significant limitations. Some of these are listed in Table 1 and discussed in detail below.

Limited Flexibility

Endovascular stents for coronary use must be highly flexible to negotiate tortuous, diseased arteries. Limited flexbility restricts the use of currently available stents to carefully selected patients. Articulated stent designs [45] and modified delivery systems have improved deployment success. With careful patient selection, deployment success by highly skilled operators exceeds 90% [46]. However, considering the potential complications from unsuccessful deployment (vessel trauma, inaccurate placement, and stent embolization), success rates for all operators must be very high. Further improvements in stent flexibility, without sacrificing mechanical performance, are needed.

Compliance Mismatch

Mismatch between the relatively inflexible stend and highly compliant coronary artery may result in continuous stress on the vessel wall. Excessive continuous lateral expansile force could cause thinning of the vessel wall. Chronic irritation produced by relatively noncompliant stent ends may induce excessive intimal hyperplasia at the stent/artery juncture. This has resulted in development of restenotic lesions in some patients receiving stents. This problem appears greater if multiple (tandem) stents are placed [44].

Thrombosis

Acute thrombosis has been a problem with all stents that are currently under investigation. Multicomponent anticoagulation and antiplatelet regimens, including heparin, coumadin, dextran, dipyridamole, and aspirin, reduce but do not eliminate this problem. These required regimens result in a significant incidence of hemorrhage and mandate further careful patient selection. Patients at risk for bleeding must be excluded from stent treatment.

Intimal Hyperplasia and Restenosis

Intimal hyperplasia appears to be a consistent response to any type of intravascular trauma. All stents induce intimal hyperplasia, even in non-atherogenic animal models. While some intimal proliferation is desirable to cover stent struts, excessive proliferation may compromise the vessel lumen. Restenosis remains a significant problem after stenting. While some lesions recur at the site of the original plaque, other de novo lesions appear to have been induced by the stent. These tend to occur at stent/artery junctures or at stent articulations, where chronic compliance mismatch (see above) may stimulate continued smooth muscle cell proliferation and migration. Because chronic irritation may occur with these permanent devices, the familiar 6-month risk period for restenosis following conventional angioplasty may not apply. Long-term (>1 year) catheterization follow-up is not yet available to assess the significance of this potential problem.

Vessel Wall Thinning

Chronic outward radial force creates the potential for thinning of the medial smooth muscle layer. This may particularly be a problem with excessively stiff or overexpanded stents. While metallic stents may induce medial thinning [47], in short-term follow-up ectasia, aneurysm formation, and vessel rupture have not been reported. The long-term fate of vessels containing permanent metal prostheses is unknown.

Balloon Rupture

Many metallic stents are deployed using balloon catheters. Wire imperfections, stent deformity, or loose wire terminations create the potential for balloon perforation. This could produce pin-hole leaks or balloon rupture, rusulting in significant coronary trauma or difficulties with proper stent deployment.

Migration and Embolization

Accurate placement of any stainless steel stent is hampered by their limited radiopacity. In addition, some balloon-expandable stents recoil as much as 15% after balloon deflation [48]. These features create the potential for improper stent sizing, which could result in stent migration after placement. Even in the hands of very skilled operators, some attempted stent placements are unsuccessful. With removal of the delivery system the stent may become dislodged, and stent embolization has been reported. The limited radiopacity of these devices makes location or retrieval very difficult.

Metallic Corrosion/Toxicity

Metallic prostheses may fail in two ways: The implant can fracture, or it can corrode, releasing potentially toxic substances. Chronic tensile stresses imposed on the stent by repeated flexing during cardiac contraction may result in stress-corrosion cracking [49], leading to accelerated corrosion and potential device failure. Two metallic sufaces in contact may undergo fretting corrosion. Tissues adjacent to stainless steel implants in humans display three types of intracellular inclusions [50]. One type of deposit appears to be hemosiderin. Similar deposits have been reported after intra-coronary stent implantation in dogs [47].

Permanent Foreign Body

Perhaps the most important limitation of metallic stents is their permanent nature. To date, stents in patients for up to 3 years have not been problematic. However, prediction of the long-term consequence of these devices is impossible. The potential for ectasia, aneurysm, perforation, and restenosis has been discussed.

The two processes treated with stents, acute occlusion and restenosis, occur shortly after angioplasty. Once tacked to the vessel wall, an intimal flap responsible for acute occlusion probably heals within several days. Restenosis appears to be rare after 6 months, and the cellular events that generate this process are most active in the first 2 weeks. Unfortunately, the only devices currently available to treat these temporary problems are permanent.

Ideal Stent Design

Sigwart's landmark report of intracoronary use of a stent in humans [51] created immediate enthusiasm for their potential impact on coronary disease. Several successful stent prototypes now exist, and modifications are being made as our understanding of the limitations of these devices evolves. Vigorous efforts have been directed at conceptualizing, designing, and constructing the ideal stent. From our present understanding of stents, we can conceptualize features of the "ideal stent" (Table 2).

Highly flexible stents would result in easier, less traumatic, and consistently successful implantations. The improved flexibility reduces com-

Table 2. Characteristics of the ideal stent

Excellent axial flexibility
Adequate radial (hoop) strength
Nonthrombogenic
Biocompatible
Easily deployable
Radiopaque
Capable of drug or cell delivery
Degradable

pliance mismatch within the vessel, resulting in less juncture restenosis and reducing long-term complications. The stent must retain adequate radial (hoop) strength to perform its mechanical function and resist vasospasm. While any foreign body in the vascular system is inherently thrombogenic, materials with favorable surface properties, modifications, or drug releasing capability should be sought. Use of stents as a vehicle for drug delivery may ultimately be their greatest utility (see below). Considering what we know about the processes that complicate angioplasty, we might envision an ideal stent that is easily and accurately deployed, releases drugs capable of resisting thrombosis and limiting smooth muscle cell proliferation, then degrades to nontoxic products for absorption.

Duke Bioabsorbable Stent

As a result of these ideal design characteristics, we have endeavored to develop a bioabsorbable stent with drug delivery capability. Facets of this development include polymer selection, stent mechanical design, experimental deployments in animal models, and ultimately clinical testing in humans.

Material Selection

Numerous characteristics must be considered in the selection of a suitable material for bioabsorbable stent development (Table 3). While many bioabsorbable polymers fashioned into fibers have excellent tensile strength (for use as bioabsorbable suture), their mechanical characteristics do not yield stents with suitable radial strength.

The polymer and its degradation products must be entirely biocompatible. Degradation should occur within a desired time frame, probably in 3–12 months. Ideally the material would retain its mechanical strength until the lesion fully heals, then degrade and absorb. The ability to modify

Table 3. Desirable characteristics of bioabsorbable stent materials

---

Excellent mechanical properties
Retention of mechanical properties in vivo
Biocompatible
Nontoxic degradation products
Desirable degradation rate and pattern
Modifiable degradation rate
Not altered by sterilization
Capable of drug delivery

---

the degradation rate and pattern through variations in polymer preparation allows the tailoring of stents to fit different clinical needs. The mechanical and degradation characteristics of the polymer must not be negatively affected by sterilization processes. Finally, the polymer should be suitable to function as a local drug delivery vehicle without serious compromise of its mechanical performance.

After experimenting with several polymers, we found poly-L-lactide (PLLA) suitable for further investigation. With special processing, the polymer yields fibers with excellent mechanical characteristics that are maintained in an aqueous environment at 37°C. Extensive in vivo experience for other applications has shown it to be biocompatible in animal models [52, 53]. It is slowly hydrolyzed, ultimately to CO_2, and excreted via the lungs. PLLA degrades very slowly in subcutaneous and intramuscular implants. No loss of tensile strength occurs after 5 months. Nine months after implantation the fiber retains approximately 75% of its original tensile strength. Microscopic examination of the fiber surface at this point shows no morphologic change [53].

Copolymers of L- and D, L-lactide degrade more quickly [54]. Surgical rods constructed from poly-D-lactide have been used to reduce mandibular fractures in dogs. After 6 weeks the rod surface appeared worm eaten; at 3 months this had progressed, and at 8 months the rods had virtually disappeared [55]. The degradation time in arterial implants has not been reported. Combinations of L- and D,L-polylactide or physicochemical alterations of PLLA would allow the degradation time of this polymer to be adjusted to fit the clinical need. We are currently investigating the degradation rates and retention of mechanical properties at various intervals after implantation of poly-L-lactide stents in animals.

Stent Design

Design selection for a stent requires consideration of radial and shear strength, method of delivery, flexibility, profile, and surface area. We have designed a stent woven in a diamond-braided pattern from 8 strands of

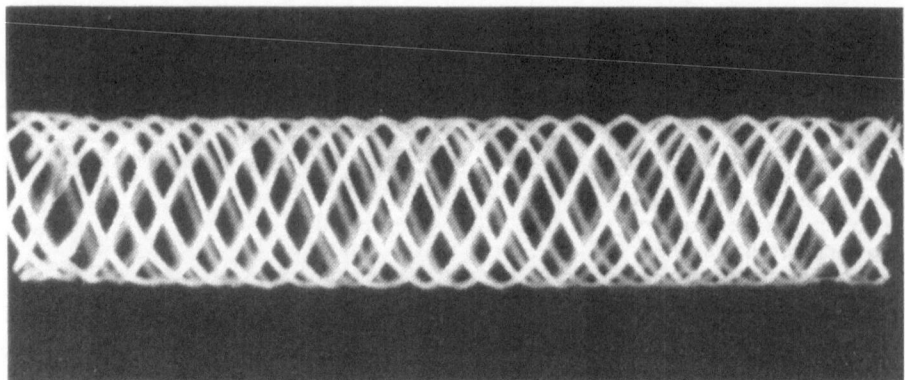

Fig. 1. Prototype of the Duke bioabsorbable stent. Bioabsorbable fibers are woven into a diamond-braided pattern, which allows the stent to assume a low profile when elongated and self-expand when delivered. (Reprinted from [42] with permission)

a highly specialized polymer that includes PLLA [56]. The stent can be elongated to assume a low profile for loading into a deployment apparatus (Fig. 1). At the site of deployment, the stent is extruded from the deployment catheter and self-expands to about the vessel wall. The stent is highly flexible and a modest surface area avoids excessive thrombosis and side branch obstruction.

In a recent abstract, results of crush pressure analysis of the Duke stent was reported [57]. A pressurized, temperature-controlled water jacket system was designed to measure the stent's ability to resist crush deformation. Studies using this device demonstrated the importance of testing polymers during exposure to warm, aqueous conditions for extended periods of time. The Duke stent retained the ability to resist crush pressures of 800–1000 mmHg for a prolonged period of time. This strength should far exceed the pressure generated by an artery in spasm [58, 59].

Experimental Deployments

In another recent abstract, initial in vivo results were reported [56]. Five stents were implanted in canine femoral arteries percutaneously. All dogs received heparin at the time of implantation but were subsequently treated with aspirin alone. The dogs were followed angiographically and harvested for pathology after a period of 2 h ($n = 1$), 1 week ($n = 1$), 2 weeks ($n = 2$), and 12 weeks ($n = 1$). All 5 stents remained patent. No inflammatory response was seen, and no significant thrombus was present. Endothelialization of the stent had occurred by 2 weeks.

Stents for Drug Delivery

Despite many improvements in angioplasty and development of new coronary microsurgical techniques, restenosis remains a major limitation to the ultimate success of any coronary intervention. Numerous trials using systemic therapy have failed to identify any agent capable of significantly reducing restenosis [24–35]. Endovascular stents may reduce this problem but clearly will not eliminate it. Thrombosis of stents has necessitated aggressive anticoagulation regimens associated with increased morbidity and variable success. Thus these two major problems, thrombosis and restenosis, remain unresolved with systemic drug therapy.

Heparin bonding techniques used for other prostheses may be adaptable to metallic stents. This may reduce, but not obviate, the need for anticoagulant therepy and is unlikely to have a significant impact on restenosis [60]. Subjecting the patient to potentially toxic systemic therapy, to treat a 1 or 2 cm diseased segment, is inefficient and potentially harmful.

A means of sustained local drug delivery at the site of arterial injury is needed. Bioabsorbable stents appear ideally suited. The stent is delivered at the time of angioplasty, which is clearly when the restenosis process begins [61–63]. The stent would perform the mechanical functions that make all stents attractive. Immediate release of antiplatelet, anticoagulant, or thrombolytic agents could simultaneously prevent thrombosis and limit restenosis. Sustained release of agents capable of stimulating reendothelialization and/or inhibiting smooth muscle cell proliferation and migration could temper the overzealous reparative process of restenosis.

Stents for Endothelial Cell Delivery

The explosion of knowledge of basic cellular processes generated by the field of molecular biology is now being applied to cardiovascular medicine [64]. An excellent example of the clinical use of recombinant DNA technology is the availability of r-tPA for the treatment of patients with acute myocardial infarction. The application of this technology to the problem of thrombosis and restenosis is an active area of research [65]. Dichek et al. [66], in a series of in vitro experiments, placed genetically modified cells (transformed to secrete r-tPA) on metallic stents and demonstrated that these cells could remain attached and secretory after balloon dilatation of the stent. Wilson et al. [67] showed that endothelial cells genetically transformed in vitro could survive on Dacron grafts in canine carotid arteries and secrete their indicator protein (β-galactosidase) for 5 weeks postimplantation. In addition, in vivo gene transfection using a retroviral vector or liposomes has now been reported [68]. Recombinant gene expression (β-galactosidase) occurred for 5 months and was limited to the site of transfection.

Bioabsorbable stents could serve as an excellent vehicle for delivery of genetically altered endothelial cells. These cells could adhere to the stent surface or be placed in surface variegations. After stent deployment, the endothelial cells would proliferate, rapidly covering the stent, and locally release the desired agent. Endothelialization could potentially occur even faster if the stent releases an endothelial cell mitogen (e.g., basic fibroblast growth factor [69]). The stent could then be absorbed, leaving a monolayer of pharmacologically active endothelial cells, with no residual foreign body.

References

1. Dotter CT (1969) Transluminally-placed coilspring endarterial tube grafts: long-term patency in canine popliteal artery. Invest Radiol 4:327–332
2. Grüntzig AR, Senning A, Siegenthaler WE (1979) Nonoperative dilation of coronary artery stenosis: percutaneous transluminal coronary angioplasty. N Engl J Med 301:61–68
3. Ellis SG, Topol EJ (1989) Intracoronary stents: will they fulfill their promise as an adjunct to angioplasty? J Am Coll Cardiol 13:1425–1430
4. Block PC (1984) Mechanism of transluminal angioplasty. Am J Cardiol 53:69C–72C
5. Cowley MJ, Dorros G, Kelsey, van Roden K, Detre KM (1984) Acute coronary events associated with percutaneous transluminal coronary angioplasty. Am J Cardiol 53:12C–16C
6. Bredlau CE, Roubin GS, Leimgruber PP et al. (1985) In-hospital morbidity and mortality in patients undergoing elective coronary angioplasty. Circulation 72: 1044–1052
7. Detre K, Holubkov R, Kelsey S et al. (1988) Percutaneous transluminal coronary angioplasty in 1985–86 and 1977–81. N Engl J Med 318:265–270
8. McBride W, Lange RA, Hillis DL (1988) Restenosis after successful coronary angioplasty: pathology and prevention. N Engl J Med 318:1734–1737
9. Ernest SM, Feltz TA, Bal ET et al. (1987) Long term angiographic follow up, cardiac events and survival in patients undergoing percutaneous transluminal coronary angioplasty. Br Heart J 57:220–225
10. Roubin GS, King SB, Douglas JS Jr (1987) Restenosis after percutaneous transluminal coronary angioplasty: the Emory University Hospital experience. Am J Cardiol 60:39B–44B
11. Holmes DR Jr, Vliestra RE, Smith HC et al. (1984) Restenosis after percutaneous transluminal coronary angioplasty (PTCA): a report from the PTCA registry of the National Heart, Lung, and Blood Institute. Am J Cardiol 53:77C–81C
12. Pepine CJ, Hirshfeld JW, MacDonald RG et al. (1990) A controlled trial of corticosteroids to prevent restenosis after coronary angioplasty. Circulation 81: 1753–1761
13. Potkin BN, Roberts WC (1988) Effects of percutaneous transluminal coronary angioplasty on atherosclerotic plaques and relation of plaque composition and arterial size to outcome. Am J Cardiol 62:41
14. Ip JH, Fuster V, Badimon L et al. (1990) Syndromes of accelerated atherosclerosis: role of vascular injury and smooth muscle proliferation. J Am Coll Cardiol 15: 1667–1687

15. Blackshear JL, O'Callaghan WG, Califf RM (1987) Medical approaches to prevention of restenosis after coronary angioplasty. J Am Coll Cardiol 9:834
16. Webster MW, Chesebro JH, Heras M et al. (1990) Effect of balloon inflation on smooth muscle cell proliferation in the porcine carotid artery (abstract). J Am Coll Cardiol 15:165A
17. Meier B, Gruentzig AR, King SB III et al. (1984) Higher balloon dilatation pressure in coronary angioplasty. Am Heart J 107:619–622
18. Quigley PJ, Kereiakes DJ, Abbottsmith CW et al. (1989) Prolonged autoperfusion angioplasty: immediate clinical outcome and angiographic follow-up (abstract). J Am Coll Cardiol 13:155A
19. Jenkins RD, Safian RD, Dear WE et al. (1990) Laser balloon angioplasty for unstable ischemic syndromes (abstract). J Am Coll Cardiol 15:245A
20. Hinohara T, Rowe M, Sipperly ME et al. (1990) Restenosis following directional coronary atherectomy of native coronary arteries (abstract). J Am Coll Cardiol 15:196A
21. Rogers PJ, Garratt KN, Kaufmann UP et al. (1990) Restenosis after atherectomy versus PTCA: initial experience (abstract). J Am Coll Cardiol 15:197A
22. Ghazzal ZM, Ba'albaki HA, Sewell CW (1990) Restenosis following coronary atherectomy; angiographic follow-up and pathologic correlates (abstract). J Am Coll Cardiol 15:57A
23. Sketch MH Jr, O'Neill WW, Tcheng JE et al. (1990) Early and late outcome following coronary transluminal extraction-endarterectomy: a multicenter experience (abstract). Circulation 82 [Suppl III]:III-310
24. Thornton MA, Gruentzig AR, Hollman J et al. (1984) Coumadin and aspirin in prevention of recurrence after transluminal coronary angioplasty: a randomized study. Circulation 69:721–727
25. White CW, Knudson M, Schmidt D et al. (1987) Ticlopidine Study Group: neither ticlopidine nor aspirin-dipyridamole prevents restenosis post PTCA: results from a randomized placebo-controlled multicenter trial (abstract). Circulation 76 [Suppl IV]: IV-213
26. Mufson L, Black A, Roubin G et al. (1988) A randomized trial of aspirin in PTCA: effect of high vs low dose aspirin on major complications and restenosis (abstract). J Am Coll Cardiol 11:236A
27. Schanzenbacher P, Grimmer M, Maisch B, Kochsiek K (1988) Effect of high dose and low dose aspirin on restenosis after primary successful angioplasty (abstract). Circulation 78 [Suppl II]:II-99
28. Slack OD, van Tassel J, Orr CM et al. (1987) Can fish oil supplement minimize restenosis after percutaneous transluminal coronary angioplasty? (abstract). J Am Coll Cardiol 9:64A
29. Milner MR, Gallino RA, Leffingwell A et al. (1988) High kose Omega-3 fatty acid supplementation reduces clinical restenosis after coronary angioplasty (abstract). Circulation 78:II-634
30. Grigg LE, Kay TW, Valentine PA et al. (1989) Determinants of restenosis and lack of effect of dietary supplementation with eicosapentaenoic acid on the incidence of coronary artery restenosis after angioplasty. J Am Coll Cardiol 13:665–672
31. Reis GS, Sipperly ME, Boucher TM et al. (1988) Results of a randomized double-blind placebo-controlled trial of fish oil for prevention of restenosis after PTCA (abstract). Circulation 78 [Suppl II]:II-291
32. Corcos T, David PR, Val PG et al. (1985) Failure of diltiazem to prevent restenosis after percutaneous transluminal coronary angioplasty. Am Heart J 109:926–931
33. Whitworth HB, Roubin GS, Hollman J et al. (1986) Effect of nidedipine on recurrent stenosis after percutaneous transluminal coronary angioplasty. J Am Coll Cardiol 8:1271–1276
34. Klein W, Eber B, Fluch N, Dusleag J (1989) Ketanserin prevents acute occlusion but not restenosis after PTCA (abstract). J Am Coll Cardiol 13:44A

35. Ellis SG, Roubin GS, Wilentz J et al. (1989) Effect of 18- to 24-hour heparin administration for prevention of restenosis after uncomplicated coronary angioplasty. Am Heart J 117:777–782
36. Sigwart U, Urban P, Golf S et al. (1988) Emergency stenting for acute occlusion after coronary balloon angioplasty. Circulation 78:1121–1127
37. Intracoronary stenting for acute closure following percutaneous transluminal angioplasty (PTCA) (1988) (abstract). Circulation 78 [Suppl II]:II-407
38. Sigwart U, Kaufman U, Goy J et al. (1988) Prevention of coronary restenosis by stenting. Eur Heart J 9 [Suppl C]:31–37
39. Puel J, Juilliere Y, Bertrand ME et al. (1988) Early and late assessment of stenosis geometry after coronary arterial stenting. Am J Cardiol 61:546–563
40. Serruys PW, Juilliere Y, Bertrand ME et al. (1988) Additional improvement of stenosis geometry in human coronary arteries by stenting after balloon dilatation. Am J Cardiol 61:71G–76G
41. Palmaz JC, Windeler SA, Garcia F et al. (1986) Balloon expandable intraluminal grafting of atherosclerotic rabbit aortas. Radiology 160:723–726
42. Stack RS, Califf RM, Phillips A et al. (1988) Interventional cardiac catheterization at Duke Medical Center: new interventional technology. Am J Cardiol [Suppl F, part II]:3F–24F
43. King SB III (1989) Vascular stents and atherosclerosis. Circulation 79:460–462
44. Ellis SG, Savage M, Baim D et al. (1990) Intracoronary stenting to prevent restenosis: preliminary results of a multicenter study using the Palmaz-Schatz stent suggest benefit in selected high risk patients (abstract). J Am Coll Cardiol 15 [Suppl A]:118A
45. Ellis SG (1990) The Palmaz-Schatz stent: potential coronary applications. In: Topol EJ (ed) Textbook of interventional cardiology. Saunders, Philadelphia, pp 623–632
46. Fajadet JC, Marco J, Cassagneau BG et al. (1990) Balloon expandable intracoronary stents: analysis of complications in a consecutive series of 160 patients (abstract). Circulation 82 [Suppl III]:III-539
47. Schatz RA, Palmaz JC, Tio FO et al. (1987) Balloon-expandable intracoronary stents in the adult dog. Circulation 76:450–457
48. Roubin GS, King SB III, Douglas JS Jr et al. (1990) Intracoronary stenting during percutaneous transluminal coronary angioplasty. Circulation 81 [Suppl IV]:IV-92–100
49. Hench LL, Ethridge EC (1982) Biomaterials. An interfacial approach. Academic, New York, pp 21–35
50. Winter GD (1974) Tissue reactions to metallic wear and corrosion products in human patients. J Biomed Mater Res Symp 5:11–26
51. Sigwart U, Puel J, Mirkovitch V et al. (1987) Intravascular stents to prevent occlusion and restenosis after transluminal angioplasty. N Engl J Med 316:701–706
52. Kulkarni RK, Pani KC, Neuman C et al. (1966) Polylactic acid for surgical implants. Arch Surg 93:839–843
53. Jamshidi K, Hyon SH, Nakamura T et al. (1986) In vitro and in vivo degradation of poly-L-lactide fibers. In: Christel P et al. (eds) Biological and biomechanical performance of biomaterials. Elsevier, Amsterdam, pp 227–232
54. Hutchinson FG, Furr BJA (1989) Biodegradable polymers for controlled release of peptides and proteins. In: Roerdink FHD, Kroon AM (eds) Drug carrier systems. John Wiley, New York, pp 111–129
55. Kulkarni RK, Moore EG, Hefyeli AF, Leonard F (1971) Biodegradable poly(lactic acid) polymers. J Biomed Mater Res 5:169–181
56. Chapman GD, Gammon RS, Bauman RB et al. (1990) A bioabsorbable stent: initial experimental results (abstract). Circulation 82 [Suppl III]:III-72
57. Howell ST, Walker WF, Stack RS, Clark HG (1990) Biodegradable intravascular stents: investigation of material properties. 16th annual meeting of the Society of Biomaterials, Charleston, p 29
58. Dobrin PB (1973) Isometric and isobaric contraction of carotid arterial smooth muscle. Am J Physiol 225:659–663

59. Cox RH (1975) Arterial wall mechanics and composition and the effects of smooth muscle activation. Am J Physiol 229:807–812
60. Cavender JB, Anderson P, Roubin GS (1990) The effects of heparin bonded tantalum stents on thrombosis and neointimal proliferation (abstract). Circulation 82 [Suppl III]:III-541
61. Grunwald J, Haudenschild CC (1984) Intimal injury in vivo activates vascular smooth muscle cell migration and explant outgrowth in vitro. Arteriosclerosis 4:183–188
62. Clowes AW, Clowes MM (1986) Kinetics of cellular proliferation after arterial injury. Circ Res 58:839–845
63. Steele PM, Chesebro JH, Stanson AW et al. (1985) Balloon angioplasty. Natural history of the pathophysiological response to injury in a pig model. Circ Res 57: 105–112
64. Chien KR, Knowlton KU (1989) Cardiovascular molecular biology: introduction to the series. Circulation 80:219–233
65. Swain JL (1989) Gene therapy. A new approach to the treatment of cardiovascular disease. Circulation 80:1495
66. Dicheck DA, Neville RF, Zwiebel JA et al. (1989) Seeding of intravascular stents with genetically engineered endothelial cells. Circulation 80:1347–1353
67. Wilson JM, Birinyi LK, Salomon RN et al. (1989) Implantation of vascular grafts lined with genetically modified endothelial cells. Science 244:1344–1346
68. Nabel EG, Plautz G, Nabel GJ (1990) Site-specific gene expression in vivo by direct gene transfer into the arterial wall. Science 249:1285–1288
69. Gospodarowicz D Biological activity in vivo and in vitro of pituitary and brain fibroblast growth factor. In: Ford RJ, Maizel AL (eds) Mediators in cell growth and differentiation. Raven, New York, pp 109–134

Conclusion

U. SIGWART[1]

Coronary Stents: Will They Survive?

Early concepts of endovascular support devices [1, 2] have received great attention since the first human implants were performed in 1986 [3]. Five years later, the first generation of vascular stents can be looked upon with constructive scepticism mixed with guarded optimism for future developments.

The Problem of Stent Thrombosis

Between 1986 and 1991 all clinically used stents were made of metal. Different surgical steel alloys with varying physical characteristics, making them either plastically deformable or springy have been used. Also nickel titanium with or without memory characteristics, or tantalum alloys with high radiopacity have been tried. All these metals suffer from undesirable surface characteristics, including electrical charges, which promote thrombosis.

Thrombosis has become the Achilles' heel of all first generation stents. The early optimism reflected by the lack of severe anticoagulation recommendations for the post-implant period was rapidly reversed after numerous thrombotic complications and high rates of restenosis were recognised. After these sobering observations, even the most optimistic stent investigators have changed their regimen to a now generally accepted combination of antiplatelet compounds together with warfarin; only the duration of treatment varies somewhat from centre to centre, in general it is maintained for the first 3–6 months. During the implantation period, all stent investigators give high doses of heparin together with dextran. This practice has shifted the problem away from early stent thrombosis towards local bleeding complications at the puncture site. For all balloon expandable and self-

[1] Royal Brompton National Heart and Lung Hospitals, Sydney Street, London SW3 6NP, Great Britain

Coronary Stents
Edited by U. Sigwart and G.I. Frank
© Springer-Verlag Berlin Heidelberg 1992

expanding metal stents, local bleeding complications can be expected in at
least one in ten procedures.

Two potential approaches to these problems are being contemplated:
either reduction of stent thrombogenicity or new approaches to haemostasis
at the puncture site despite full anticoagulation. The latter approach is likely
to yield immediate success by new technologies using means of favouring
healing of the femoral artery puncture site, the former will require totally
new materials, new stent designs and local drug delivery systems.

Local haemostasis despite full anticoagulation can be obtained using
puncture site sealing with collagen plugs [4]. In a series of 50 patients on full
anticoagulation with heparin (mean activated clotting time 417 s), we tried
to seal the arterial puncture site with collagen plugs immediately after
the procedure. There were two procedural failures, probably secondary to
early learning experience and one case of leg ischaemia; a later surgical
intervention revealed severe atherosclerosis of the iliac artery but no complications attributed to the sealing procedure. Prolonged bleeding was
observed only in two patients, none requiring surgical intervention or
transfusions.

Prolonged local compression has equally helped to deal with the problem of puncture site bleeding. A belt compression device with a transparent
air cushion placed over the puncture site can be used to generate pressures
high enough to prevent bleeding but low enough to allow unimpeded
femoral artery blood flow. This FemoStop compressor permits excellent
monitoring of the puncture site and is comfortable enough to be left in place
for extended periods. A combination of enhancement of clotting by collagen
together with prolonged air cushion compression may well be the solution to
puncture site bleeding after stenting despite full anticoagulation.

Modification of stents, making them less thrombogenic or not at all
thrombogenic is a much more difficult task. Alteration of the strut surface
by mechanical or chemical polishing has not yielded reproducible reduction
in stent thrombosis. Coating with biocompatible polymers known to be somewhat platelet repellent has produced conflicting data [5]. Despite more
than 50% platelet deposition reduction measured with indium-111 oxine in
baboon shunts, no clinically reproducible advantage of such surface treatment could be seen. Research is being directed towards the role of surface chemistry, surface structure and surface charge in order to minimise
thrombotic phenomenon. To date it is not clear whether such effort is
justified. The role of platelets in the healing process of vascular injury
needs to be studied in much more detail. Platelets, with their propensity to
stimulate smooth muscle cell growth, may play an important positive role in
the initial phase of the repair process, including a beneficial, controlled
neointimal ingrowth. Therefore, rough surfaces may well have advantages
over platelet repellent surfaces, provided single layers of platelet deposition
can be achieved (Fig. 1).

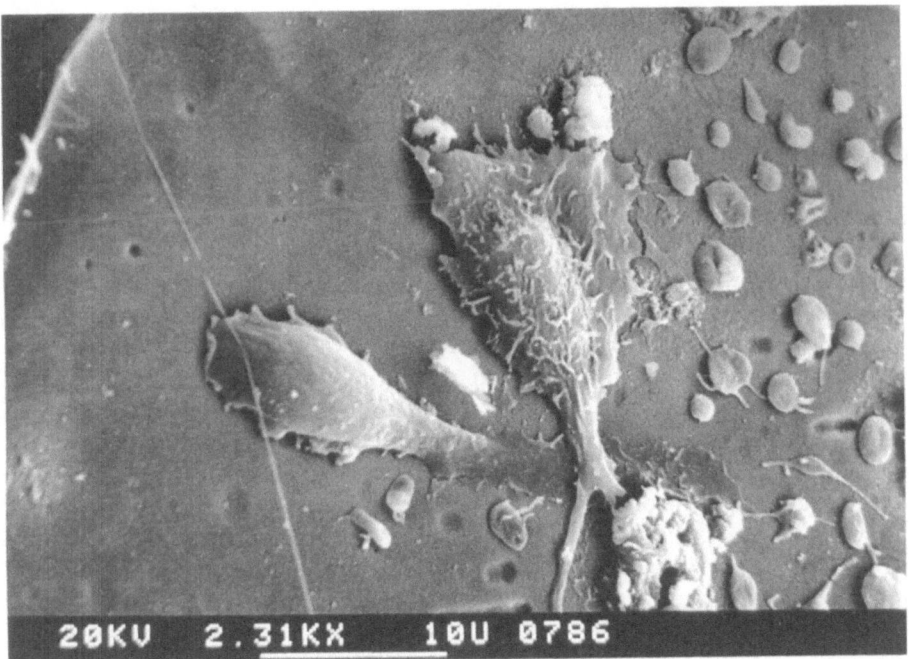

Fig. 1. Nontreated, relatively rough metal surface on a stent implanted for 1 week in a rabbit aorta. Apart from platelets and macrophages smooth muscle cells may adhere to this surface *without* interposition of significant thrombosis

Total suppression of platelet adhesion may be realised using biologically active substances. Heparin and heparin derivatives have been tried as well as hirudin and synthetic antithrombins. These substances supplied in relatively high concentration inhibite platelet deposition, thrombosis and, possibly by virtue of suppression of platelet deposition, smooth muscle cell proliferation. Coating of currently used metal stents with these substances poses a number of problems. Firstly, binding of biologically active substances to metal surfaces is difficult and, secondly, controlled release is not easily achieved. Therefore matrix-controlled release systems are favoured for local drug delivery. They consist of a supporting structure composed of polymer material functioning as a skeleton which is surrounded by pockets filled with drugs. The pockets may be connected by pores. In order to be released, the drug must traverse this complex network. This requires entry of fluid and diffusion of the drug through the network of channels. The molecular mass of the drug and the size of the channels determine the dilution pattern. Using matrix-controlled release systems, thrombosis and smooth muscle proliferation can be effectively inhibited [6]. Whether these techniques have any benefit in the clinical setting by reducing the amount of thrombosis and the number of restenoses remains to be demonstrated.

The concept, however, of administering antithrombotic substances locally is attractive. Suppression of thrombosis by systemic administration of heparin, hirudin or other newer synthetic antithrombins requires concentrations that may induce systemic complications. Systemic use of new compounds like synthetic antithrombins have been reported to be beneficial in suppressing stent thrombosis [5]. et al. High concentrations in the region of interests without significant systemic effects are of course desirable. The choice of material (heparin, hirudin, antithrombins etc.) is probably less important than the precise release mechanism and the concentration in loco.

It is doubtful whether cell seeding with endothelial cells, capable of enhanced recombinant tissue-type plasminogen activator (t-PA) production will be the answer to the problem of thrombosis. Stent technology is a compromise between biological requirements and practical aspects; cell seeding requires extremely delicate handling, involves problems of storage and preparation, and is not free from danger of infection [7].

In summary, thrombosis remains the main issue in stenting. Systemic anticoagulation is not effective enough despite improvements in puncture site haemostasis. In situ antithrombotic treatment may become the method of choice if reliable drug delivery systems can be built.

Structural Support and Flow Patterns

Stents are supposed to provide structural support to the artery; the amount of radial force needed to prevent recoil and intrusion of material is difficult to assess. It is not known either whether such structural support is needed for very short or long periods and whether after healing of the actual angioplasty injury such support is no longer useful. The optimal spacing between filaments equally requires further research.

After implantation of balloon expandable or self-expanding stents into coronary arteries in animals, the rigidity of these devices becomes immediately evident when palpating the outside of the heart, where the unstented parts are soft and pliable and the stented segments stand out by their hardness. In diseased human coronary arteries this difference is less impressive since the arteries themselves are quite rigid. To support coronary dissections very little radial pressure is needed; to counter-balance elastic recoil in severely fibrotic arterial disease important radial forces are needed. Ideally, stents with different radial compliance might be employed for different disease states.

Stents with little resistance to radial force can be built with lesser filament diameter and lower profile. This consideration becomes important in view of the turbulence generated by each individual strut (Fig. 2). Clinically used stents have filament diameters varying between 60 and 150 μ in thickness. In small diameter arteries the wire thickness plays an important

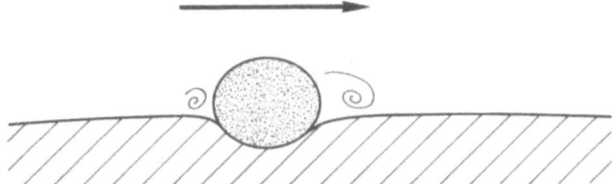

Fig. 2. Cross-section through a stent wire and the adjacent artery. Note the potential for turbulence created by the uncovered stent wire

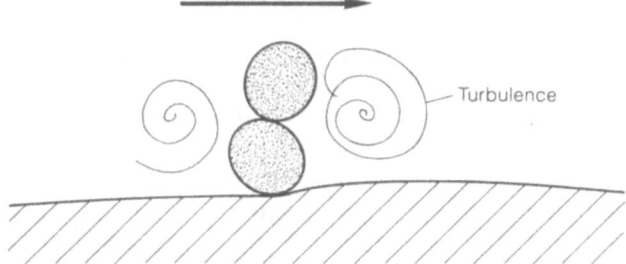

Fig. 3. Wire crossings may create even greater turbulence

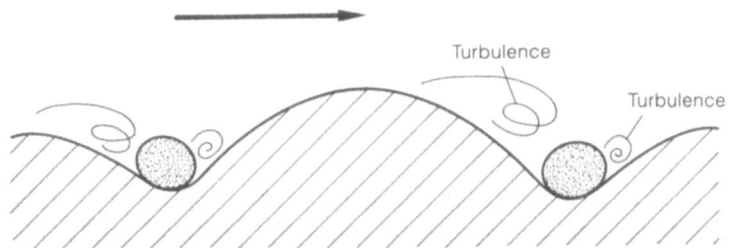

Fig. 4. Stent wires exert pressure on the arterial wall only where they are in contact with the tissue. The uncovered holes between the wires protrude into the arterial lumen, thus creating important trubulence

role, particularly, as in case of the self-expanding stent, if wire crossings exist (Fig. 3). Turbulence is known to be a precipitating factor of thrombosis and atherosclerosis. Therefore, low profile struts appear desirable and the stent filament diameter should be reduced to the absolute minimum needed for adequate support of the artery. Stent wires with $150\,\mu$ diameter in 3 mm diameter arteries must create undesirable turbulence. In addition to the turbulence created by the struts themselves, stents produce further turbulence by indenting the artery wherever wire inhibits elastic recoil. The

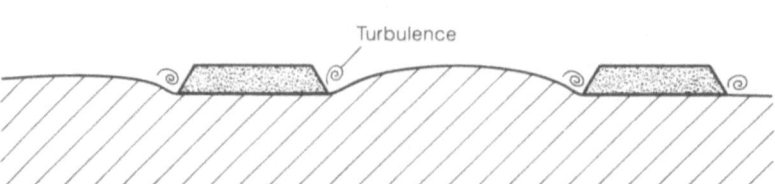

Fig. 5. A low profile optimally spaced stent may diminish the stasis and turbulence significantly

non-supported vessel segments therefore bulge into the lumen and create further turbulence (Fig. 4). Turbulence produces stasis, platelet aggregation, deposition of other blood elements, thrombosis and smooth muscle cell proliferation. This phenomenon can easily be observed histologically in segments of animal and human speciments.

Ideally a stent should consist of a conformable elastic macroporous tube, the holes of which are small enough to guarantee a homogenous surface, large enough not to impede flow to side branches, and thin enough not to create significant turbulence (Fig. 5). These goals have to be kept in mind when contemplating concepts for new stents. Stents that have been used so far in clinical trials appear like rude devices. Apart from providing inadequate surface characteristics, their geometry is so rudimentary that a highly significant reduction in the number of restenoses appears unlikely.

Materials

The choice of materials for stents has been dictated in the past by structural characteristics, proven biocompatibility and availability. Non-metallic stents were tried as early as 1912 [1] and Dotter [2] also used plastic tubes for arterial support. Glass and ceramics, despite their attractive surface characteristics, are unsuitable because they are rigid and brittle. To date, only metal stents (nickel titanium alloys, surgical steel alloys and tantalum alloys) have been used in clinical trials. As mentioned before they all suffer from their surface characteristics as well as from the difficulty to incorporate biologically active drugs. Polymers have gained recent interest, particularly in view of local drug delivery. Early experiments with biostable polymers were disappointing but it is not known whether the surface characteristics or the flow characteristics are responsible for the massive smooth muscle cell proliferation observed with these stents [8].

Bioerodable stents with or without drug delivery systems are currently under investigation in animals. Despite the fact that the metabolism of a number of bioerodable polymers is insufficiently understood, research continues in this direction. Bioerodable stents have the advantage of permitting free access to side branches once the stent has vanished. They also allow further transluminal interventions in case of secondary disease. The choice of material is limited. The physical properties of polymers used in stents will always be measured against the standard of surgical stainless steel. Some polylactic acid compounds seem to be coming close to the strength but not to the elasticity of surgical stainless steel. Further modifications of these types of polymers as well as hybrid constructions made out of sandwich type elements are under investigation.

Stent Delivery

If stents can be made inoffensive and non-thrombogenic, promote healing and reduce restenosis, widespread application may be desirable. With a combined effort from industry and medical research, it may become possible to cover each angioplasty site with a sort of wound dressing which guarantees optimal flow, counterbalances recoil and controls endothelisation. Such extended use would require delivery systems that are not more complicated and equal in performance than the angioplasty devices currently being used.

The original delivery system for the self-expanding stent may be too complicated for widespread use. The positioning of stents with this device is quite delicate and even in experienced hands, slight variations in the final stent position may be encountered while employing the device. Also, due to the shortening fraction of self-expanding stents, the final length of the stented segment is more or less unpredictable. Delivery failure has equally been observed in several cases. For these reasons, operator friendly delivery systems allowing for extremely high precision deployment, trackability and safety are needed. The original sheath technology to protect stents from being embolised proved invaluable where the safety in rough and tortuous arterial segments is concerned. The protective sleeve withdrawal mechanism, however, is not totally foolproof; despite operator experience and patience, the release mechanism may fail in some cases. Simpler ways are now possible based on tubular sheaths without invaginating membranes. The friction between the coaxial elements can greatly be reduced with the help of lubricating substances. Instruments are now available with a diameter of 5 F which pass through any guiding catheter of 8 F.

Balloon expansion of stents is incomparably more precise than placement of self-expanding stents with conventional assistance. Metal markers defining the position and length of the stent on the delivery device are extremely helpful. Stents with no shortening during expansion can thus be deployed with better than 1 mm deployment precision. Stretchable membranes between balloon and stent matrix can be used to assure even expansion throughout the entire stent length.

Summary

Even with the first "generation" stents some vascular conditions can be treated very effectively: dissections can very well be sealed with stents, resulting in patent vessels and thus avoiding emergency surgery, embolisation of friable material can be prevented, particularly in bypass grafts, and elastic recoil in rubbery lesions is reliably counteracted. The question of restenosis, however, is still open to debate, although some studies have shown very significant reduction in restenosis. The key issue seems to be how the exaggerated repair mechanisms with its uncontrolled ingrowth of smooth muscle cells can be prevented. Many researchers are focus sing now on ways of reducing mitotic rates and counteracting growth factors generated from the traumatised arterial wall. Whether these tissue factors are the most important stimuli for hypoplasia is questionable. It may very well be that fluid dynamics are equally important. The fact that nowadays stents have not in all cases yielded satisfactory results [9] does not mean that tissue factors dominate the scene. Arteries are not static organs! Looking at the neoendothelial lining after angioplasty or after implantation of stents, one may get the impression that new cell formations are being triggered and oriented according to the blood flow. If laminar flow can be achieved through creation of a new arterial tapestry in the form of a trellis with small openings, smooth surface and extremely thin matrix, permitting orientation of the orderly cellular ingrowth but not suppressing it, the battle may be won.

References

1. Carrel A (1912) Results of the permanent intubation of the thoracic aorta. Surg Gyn Obstet 16:245–248
2. Dotter CT (1969) Transluminally placed coil spring arterial tube grafts: long term patency in canine popliteal artery. Invest Radiol 4:329–332
3. Sigwart U, Puel J, Mirkovitch V, Joffre F, Kappenberger L (1987) Intravascular stents to prevent occlusion and restenosis after transluminal angioplasty. N Engl J Med 316:701–706
4. Ernst J, Kloos R, Schrader R, Kaltenbach M, Sigwart U, Sanborn TA (1991) Immediate sealing of arterial puncture sites after catheterization and PTCA using a vascular haemostatic device with collagen: an international registry. Circulation 84 [Suppl 2]:69 (Abstract)
5. Krupski WC, Bass A, Kelly AB, Marzec UM, Hanson SR, Harker LA (1990) Heparin-resistant thrombus formation by endovascular stents in baboons. Interruption by a synthetic antithrombin. Circulation 82:570–577

6. Edelman ER, Adams DH, Karnovsky MJ (1991) Effect of controlled adventitial heparin delivery on smooth muscle cell proliferation following endothelial injury. Proc Natl Acad Sci USA 87:3773–3777
7. Dichek DA, Neville RF, Zwiebel JA, Freeman SM, Leon MB, Anderson WF (1989) Seeding of intravascular stents with genetically engineered endothelial cells. Circulation 80:1347–1353
8. Schwartz RS, Murphy JG, Edwards WD, Camrud AR, Vlietstra RE, Holmes DR (1990) Restenosis after angioplasty: a practical proliferative model in porcine coronary arteries. Circulation 82:2190–2200
9. Block PC Coronary artery stents and other endoluminal devices. N Engl J Med 324(1):52-e (editorial)

Subject Index